Soccer & Science

Editor and Series editor
Jens Bangsbo

Munksgaard

Institute of Exercise and Sport Sciences
University of Copenhagen

Copenhagen 2000

SOCCER & SCIENCE

Copyright © Institute of Exercise and Sport Sciences, University of Copenhagen

Editor: Jens Bangsbo
Series editor: Jens Bangsbo
Design and layout: Allis Skovbjerg Jepsen
Front page: Harald Giersing. Fodboldspillere. Sofus header. 1917. Aarhus Kunst-museum
Fotos: Sportsfoto. Page 16: The Arcive of National Olympic Committee and Sports Confederation of Denmark.
Printed By: Special-Trykkeriet Viborg a/s

ISBN 87 16 12348-4

Printed in Denmark 2000

Institute of Exercise and Sport Sciences
University of Copenhagen
Nørre Allé 51
DK-2200 Copenhagen

Phone: +45 35 32 08 29
Fax: +45 35 32 08 70
e-mail: IFI@ifi.ku.dk
Homepage: www.ifi.ku.dk

Content

Preface

In August 1997 the 2nd "European Congress of Sport and Exercise Science" was held in Copenhagen with more than 800 participants. The scientific programme covered all aspects of exercise and sport sciences with more than 100 invited speakers and 400 presentations. Within the theme "Science and Sport" a number of symposia covered sports from a multidiciplinary perspective. As many people have expressed an interest in this multidisciplinary approach of sport we have decided to produce a series of books on soccer, sailing, running and European diversity in sport and physical activity, respectively. We have been fortunate that so many experts have agreed to contribute to the books allowing for an integration of physiological, psychological, historical and social aspects of the sport. Each chapter in the books provides up-to-date knowledge about the topic and includes a high number of references to allow the reader to go further into depth with the subject area. It is anticipated and hoped that the books will be useful for university researchers, teachers and students as well as for interested coaches.

We will like to express our appreciation to the authors and reviewers as well as the editors for their great effort, which has enabled us to produce these informative books.

Jens Bangsbo
Series Editor

Preword

Soccer and Science covers a multidisciplinary scientific approach to the game of soccer as performance in soccer is influenced by a great variety of factors, not only related to the game on the field, but also outside of the field. Thus, physiological and nutritional aspects as well as psychological, ethical and sociological factors are included in this book. Any scientific approach has to have its foundation in the game and the authors of this book are duly selected by their combined scientific expertise and long term practical experience within soccer. The chapters are of a high scientific quality yet are written in an easily understandable manner, in order to reach also the non-scientific reader. I highly recommend that you take the time to read the chapters that cover also areas outside of your own expertise to get further insight into the complexity of the game of soccer.

I will take this opportunity to extend my gratitude to the authors and the individuals who have been involved in the reviewing of chapters in this book, Eric Dunning, Bjarne Ibsen, Birger Peitersen, Ronald Renson, Stuart Biddle and Reinhard Stelter.

I hope that you will find the book interesting and enjoy your reading!

Jens Bangsbo
Editor

List of Authors

JENS BANGSBO, Institute of Exercise and Sport Siences, University of Copenhagen, Universitetsparken 13, DK-2100 Copenhagen Ø, Denmark. Telephone: (+45) 3532 1623 Fax: (+45) 3532 1600 E-mail: JBangsbo@aki.ku.dk

ERIC DUNNING, Centre for Research into Sport and Society, University of Leicester, 14 Salisbury Road, Leicester LE1 7RQ, United Kingdom. Telephone: 0116 252 5929 E-mail: crss@le.ac.uk

YURI L. HANIN, Research Institute for Olympic Sports, Rautpohjankatu 6, 40700 Jyvaskyla, Finland. Telephone 358-14-2603-175 (or 170) Fax: 358-14-2603-171 E-mail: yhanin@kihu.jyu.fi

HAN INKLAAR, Sports Medical Center Royal Netherlands Football Association, Woudenbergsweg 56, 3707 HX Zeist, Netherlands. Telephone: 31 343 499285 Fax: 31 343 499288.

JOSEPH MAGUIRE, Department of Physical Education, Sports Science and Recreation Management, Loughborrough University, Leicestershire LE11 3TU, United Kingdom. Telephone: (+44) (0) 1509 223328 Fax: (+44) (0) 1509 223971

PER NILSSON, Stockholm Institute of Education, Department of Educational Research, P.O.Box 341 03, S-100 26 Stockholm, Sweden. Telephone: (+46) 8 737 56 11 Fax: (+46) 8 737 56 10 E-mail: per.nilsson@lhs.se

THOMAS REILLY, Research Institute for Sport and Exercise Sciences, Henry Cotton Campus, Webster Street, Liverpool L3 2ET, United Kingdom. Telephone: (+44) (0) 151 231 4324 E-mail: t.p.reilly@livjm.ac.uk

DAVID STEAD, Department of Physical Education, Sports Science and Recreation Management, Loughborrough University, Leicestershire LE11 3TU, United Kingdom. Telephone: (+44) (0) 1509 223282 Fax: (+44) (0) 1509 223971 E-mail: D.E.Stead@lboro.ac.uk

About the Authors

Eric Dunning is Emeritus Professor of Sociology at the University of Leicester and currently holds Visiting Professorships at University College Dublin and the University of Ulster at Jordanstown. He has authored and co-authored several books on the Sociology of Sport, most notably on sport and violence, and is currently working on aspects of Nazism and the Holocaust. An active footballer until his late thirties, He played for the University of Leicester from 1956 to 1961, also playing for Hayes, Oadby Town and Old Actonians.

David Stead is a lecturer in the Sociology of Sport in the Department of Physical Education, Sports Science and Recreation Management at Loughborough University, England. He entered academic life after a long career as a manager and adviser concerned with a wide range of social and cultural policy issues. This included membership of numerous governmental and non-governmental advisory bodies on sport, particularly with regard to provision for young people. More latterly, he has researched and written on globalisation and sport issues, specifically athletic labour migration. He has a particular interest in elite level sport and the personal and professional experiences of the athletes involved.

Joseph Maguire is Professor of the Sociology of Sport in the Department of Physical Education, Sports Science and Recreation Management at Loughborough University, England. He is President of the International Sociology of Sport Association. He has served on the editorial boards of a number of journals and has published extensively, including his latest work, Global SPORT. Identities Societies Civilizations (1999) Polity Press. His current research interests include sport and national identity, sport and labour migration and sport violence.

Per Nilsson is Associate Professor at Stockholm Institute of Education and Reader in Sport and Education at Stockholm University College of Physical Education. He was a visiting Professor at Cheltenham & Gloucester College of Higher Education in the autumn of 1997. Per Nilsson's main research interests circle around sport and socialisation, leisure and youth, and body and identity, and he has written a great number of articles and books on these topics. Per Nilsson is also a member of the medical subcommittee within The Swedish Football Association.

Yuri L. Hanin is a Professor and Senior Researcher at the Research Institute for Olympic Sports (KIHU), Jyväskylä, Finland. He has carried out extensive research, training, and consulting with national, international, and Olympic level teams, athletes, and coaches. He is well known as a speaker at conferences throughout Europe, USA, Canada, and Australia. His new book on „Emotions in Sports" (Human Kinetics) summarizes research findings related to optimizing sports performance. He is a recipient of the 1998 Visiting Scholar Award from the Australian College of Sport Psychologists and the 1999 Distinguished International Scholar Award from the Association for the Advancement of Applied Sport Psychology (AAASP).

Thomas Reilly is Director of the Research Institute for Sport and Exercise Sciences at Liverpool John Moores University. He acts as Chair of the International Steering Group on Science and Football and organised the 1st World Congress of Science and Football at Liverpool in 1987. He has chaired the British Olympic Association's Exercise Physiology Steering Group since 1992. He is a Fellow of the Institute of Biology and holds a D.Sc. award in chronobiology.

Jens Bangsbo is Associate Professor at the Institute of Exercise and Sport Sciences, University of Copenhagen, where he achieved his doctoral degree with the thesis „Physiology of Soccer – with a special reference to high intensity intermittent exercise". He has written more than one hundred original papers and reviews. He is the author of 12 books published in a number of different languages. He is a member of the Copenhagen Muscle Research Centre. He has received the „Biochemistry of Exercise" award. He is a member of the International Steering Group on Science and Football. He is a former professional soccer player and has played more than four hundred matches in the Danish top league as well as several matches in the Danish National team.

Han Inklaar is currently head of the Department for Sports Medicine at the Sports Medical Center of the Royal Netherlands Football Association. He is chairman of the scientific committee of the Netherlands Association for Sports Medicine. His field of interest is the epidemiology of sports injuries. In 1985 he was honoured with the Netherlands award for Sports Medicine for his study on sports injuries presented at the general practice. In the Netherlands he has written several articles and books on different topics of sports medicine.

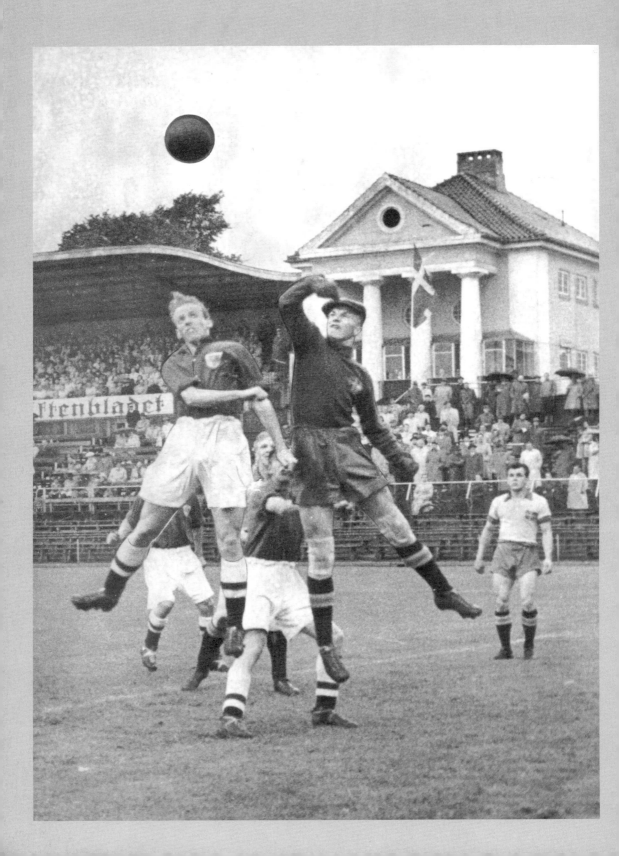

Football in the Civilizing Process

Eric Dunning

Synopsis

This chapter involves an application of Elias's theory of 'civilizing processes' in an attempt to illuminate key aspects of the early development of modern football. After an exposition of the main parameters of Elias's theory in which it is established that the theory is neither a 'unilinear' nor a 'progress' theory, there follows a description and analysis of the folk antecedents of modern football, how these came to be culturally marginalized and how prototypical versions of soccer and rugby were 'co-produced' in the status-tension-ridden social field of the English public schools. The national and international spread of these game-forms and the formation of national and international associations are then discussed. The chapter finishes with a brief diagnosis of the international popularity of soccer and why that game is associated almost universally with 'hooliganism' or spectator violence and disorder.

Introduction

The development of sport as a world phenomenon in the course of the twentieth century and its growing significance in international as well as intra-national relations is one of the prime indicators of the accelerating processes of globalization that have characterized the modern world (I include under the term, 'modern world', what has fashionably but in my view misleadingly come to be called our current, 'postmodern' era).[1] In this chapter, I shall use Elias's theory of 'civilizing processes' (6, 9) in an attempt to shed light on the early development of one of these world sports – the 'soccer' form of football. I shall also examine, less intensively, its global spread and attempt to illuminate why soccer has been more successful in diffusing internationally than the rugby and American forms of the game. Finally, I shall briefly pay attention to the related issue of why hooligan behaviour has come to occur more frequently in conjunction with soccer than with these other ludic forms. However, centrally underlying my paper will be the contention that Elias's theory of civilizing processes is a fruitful vehicle for shedding light on processes such as those connected with the development and diffusion of modern sports. Accordingly, a primary requirement for appreciating the analysis which follows is a proper understanding of what Elias's theory of civilizing processes does and does not entail.

The bedrock on which the theory of civilizing processes rests is the research-based observation, primarily established by reference to a mass of French, British, German and, to a lesser extent, Italian data, that there took place in the countries of Western Europe between the Middle Ages and the early twentieth century a refinement of social standards, together with an increase in the pressure on people to exercise stricter, more continuous self-control over their feelings and behaviour. As part of this, and of central relevance for the development of football and modern sport more generally, there occurred a tightening in the social control of violence and aggression, coupled with a long-term decline in most people's propensity for and capability of obtaining pleasure from taking part in and witnessing acts of physical aggression other than those of a relatively controlled and mimetic kind (11, 1). Psychologically, or better, at the levels of personality and habitus,[2] this entailed: (i) an advance in people's 'threshold of repugnance' regarding violence and bloodshed; and (ii) the internalization of stricter taboos on violence as part of the 'conscience' or 'superego'. Of course, to refer to these developments as a 'civilizing process' is not to make the absurd suggestion that violence in Western societies has been or ever will be totally eliminated, but rather to contend among other things that – and notwithstanding the national, class and gender differences which remain in this regard – a majority of Western people have grown more sensitive to the non-mimetic manifestations of violence and that violence in its non-mimetic forms has been increasingly privatized, ie, pushed more and more 'behind the scenes'.

Besides witnessing the global spread of sports, the twentieth century has also been a century of scientific and technological advance at a hitherto unprecedented pace and on a hitherto unprecedented scale. However, in addition it has witnessed the widespread deployment of science and technology in genocide and war. Science and technology have also come to be seen as contributing to ecological damage on a global scale. Hence, it is not perhaps surprising that many people in the West, whilst increasingly relying on science and technology in a host of obvious and less obvious ways – including in the sphere of sport – should simultaneously have come to lose the blind faith in 'progress' that was a dominant belief of their eighteenth and nineteenth century forebears. Nor is it perhaps surprising in the ideological climate of ambivalence or even outright hostility towards 'progress' that is characteristic of the present-day West, that a common gut reaction to Elias's theory is to dismiss it out of hand as an outmoded 'evolutionary' or 'progress' theory.[3] However, such a visceral reaction is premature. Let me endeavour to substantiate how and why that is the case. In order to do so, I shall have to undertake a fairly lengthy discussion of issues which are not directly connected with the development of modern sport but are nevertheless vital to a proper sociological understanding of that process.

In *The Civilizing Process,* Elias started by considering the meaning of the term 'civilization' and reached the conclusion that, since any aspect of human society and behaviour can be judged as 'civilized' or 'uncivilized', providing such a definition is a difficult if not impossible task. It is easier, said Elias, to specify the function of the term. It has come, he argued, to express the self-image of the most powerful western nations and it has acquired in that connection derogatory and racist connotations, not only in relation to what Westerners call the 'primitive' or 'barbaric' non-western societies they have conquered, colonized or otherwise subjected to domination but also in relation to 'less advanced', ie, less powerful, societies and outsider groups in the West itself. Interestingly, Elias showed how the First World War was fought by Britain and France against Germany in the name of 'civilization', and how, in the eighteenth, nineteenth and early twentieth centuries when the formerly disunited and therefore relatively weak Germans were engaged in a process of trying to catch up with their more united and powerful western neighbours, many Germans became ambivalent about the term 'civilization', preferring to express their self-image through the more particularistic concept of *Kultur,* ie, 'culture' (6, 9, 17).

A further way in which Elias sought to distance his theory from the evaluative connotations of the popular concept of civilization was by means of an explicit denial that Western societies have come to represent some kind of 'end-point' or 'pinnacle' in this regard (9: 522). People in the present-day West may consider themselves to be 'civilized' and regard Western civilization as 'complete', but whilst it can be empirically shown that they have grown *more* 'civilized' than their medieval predecessors in certain limited respects – ie, that, although there is no guarantee that such a process will continue in the future, they can be said to have undergone a 'civilizing process' in a *technical* sense – Elias was clear that present-day Westerners are far from being civilized in any absolute way and speculated that future historians may come to judge even the most civlizationally 'advanced' present-day Western societies and groups as having formed part of an 'extended Middle Ages' (6, 9) and their members as 'late barbarians' (8). The reverse side of the idea that the present-day West does not represent a 'pinnacle' of civilization according to Elias is that, with the marginal exception of the unborn and as yet unsocialized child, there is no zero-point of civilization, no absolutely uncivilized society or individual.

It is neither possible nor necessary in the context of this paper to specify in detail the entire spectrum of factual developments which Elias saw as constituting the Western European civilizing process. It is enough just to stress that he was clear, firstly about the delimitation of this process in terms of space and time, and, secondly, about the fact that, as with social developments more generally, it has been based on the inter-generational transmission of learned experiences. Hence it is reversible. At the core of Elias's explanation, lies the idea that state-formation, the unplanned or 'blind' establishment of relatively stable and secure centralized state monopolies on the major 'means of ruling' – violence and taxation – provides a key, processes in which violent 'hegemonial' or 'elimination' struggle among kings and other feudal lords were decisive. Using more conventional language what was involved was the gradual transition via competitive struggle from highly decentralized feudal states to more highly centralized dynastic states and eventually to nation-states.

According to Elias, an important corollary of this unplanned process was the gradual pacification of larger and larger spaces within each developing state. In a word, states which remained externally embattled at each stage – and it is crucial to remember that – became increasingly pacified internally. (There are signs of slight reversal of this process having occurred sine the 1960s and 1970s. (4)). In turn, domestic pacification facilitated material production, the growth of trade, an increase in the amount and circulation of money together with a growing 'monetarization' of social relations, and correlatively with all of this, a lengthening of interdependency chains, ie, a shift from bonds of interdependence which were primarily local in scope to bonds which became increasingly national and subsequently international. All of these part processes were involved in reciprocal interaction with each other. That is to say, the relationships among them cannot be described in terms of simple causes and effects.

According to Elias, the 'macrosocial' consequences of this complex of changes were principally threefold. More particularly, there took place: (i) a further augmentation of state – in the first instance given the private ownership of the means of ruling at that stage, primarily of royal – power, because tax revenues and the capacity of governments to equip standing armies increased; (ii) a progressive augmentation of the power of middle class or 'bourgeois' groups whose power and status depended primarily on relatively fluid and expandable monetary resources as opposed to the comparatively fixed resource of land; and (iii) a correlative weakening of the 'warrior aristocracy', ie of knights whose power depended fundamentally on land ownership and the force of arms. At the point where the power of these rising middle class and falling upper class groups became approximately equal, kings became able to play off one against the other and uphold a claim to 'absolute rule'.

The development of monarchical absolutism went further in France than anywhere else in Western Europe and it was in that context, according to Elias, that what he called 'the courtization of the warriors' *(die Verhöflichung der Krieger)* began most significantly to occur, ie, they began to be tamed and transformed from rough and ready 'free' or independent 'knights' into urbane and polished 'courtiers' who were dependent on the king. In Britain, by contrast, claims to absolute rule proved impossible to sustain, and monarchs were forced to share the business of ruling with parliament. Accordingly, in the British context the royal court shared its civilizing function with parliament and 'Society', the assembly of noble and untitled 'gentlemen' and 'ladies' whose 'London season' coincided more or less with when parliament met. After the eighteenth century, it also shared it with the 'public schools' [4] and the universities of Oxford and Cambridge. This overall figuration was arguably crucial to the fact that the initial development of modern sport took place in Britain. Moreover, civilizing developments in the public schools were crucial to the initial development of soccer and its split from the rugby way of playing football.

According to Elias, there were differences between the civilizing and state-formation processes of Britain and France, though in both cases, these processes were relatively continuous in the longer term (9). This contrasted markedly with German developments which were, Elias argued, more discontinuous. In Germany, a number of deep-rooted structural obstacles for a long while impeded state-centralization, the emergence of a powerful and relatively independent middle class and hence the development of more democratic values, attitudes and institutions. In fact, Germany did not become a relatively unified nation-state until 1871 and it did so through warfare under the hegemony of the militaristic Prussians. In such a context, the Germans remained subject to forms of absolutist rule until 1918 and this became deeply rooted in the habitus, conscience and traditions of a majority of German people. This helps to explain the central part played by Germany in the origins of the First and Second World Wars and the rise of Nazism and 'the Holocaust'. It also helps to explain why a cult of duelling and *Turnen,* a nationalist and militaristically orientated form of gymnastics, originated in Germany rather than forms of modern sport (10, 14). To say this is not, of course, to deny that there are elements of *Turnen* in the 'sportized' and, in that sense, non-militaristic forms of gymnastics that have been incorporated into the modern Olympic Games. But let me turn to the initial development of soccer and endeavour to show how a civilising process in Elias's technical and non-evaluative sense was involved.

The 'sportization of pastimes' (7), that is, the initial development of modern forms of sport, was a process which occurred first of all in England, and to a lesser extent in Scotland, in the eighteenth and nineteenth centuries. One of the central preconditions for its occurrence was the specific trajectory of state-formation and civilization experienced by the English, above all the high degree of autonomy enjoyed by the upper and middle classes in relation to the state. Elias (7) wrote in this connection of the 'parliamentarization of political conflict' and the 'sportization of pastimes', drawing a clear parallel between the non-violent forms of party ritual developed in parliament, that is the replacement at the level of habitus among the ruling groups who were coming to regard themselves as English 'gentlemen' of military skills by the skills of debate, rhetoric and persuasion. The 'parliamentarization of political conflict' was England's equivalent of the 'courtization of the warriors', and the 'sportization of pastimes', the emergence of the relatively non-violent and ritualized forms of play that have come to attract the label 'sports', occurred as part of it.

Another precondition for the 'sportization of pastimes' was provided by pacification under state-control, a process which, together with relative autonomy from the state, facilitated the free assembly of groups in public and the relative safety of unarmed travel around the country for purposes of leisure as well as trade. Yet another precondition was provided by the fact that the relative de-militarization of upper class male roles generated the need for an enclave where traditional forms of masculinity could be expressed in relatively non-violent forms. However, since soccer developed as a modern sport out of some of the folk-games of the Middles Ages, a useful way of shedding light on this process is by means of a comparison of the structural properties of the folk antecedents of modern football with those of their present-day equivalents. I have attempted this diagramatically in Fig. 1:

In the Middle Ages and early modern period – and this was true, not only of England but of many, if not all, continental European countries, too – people played games that they called 'football' as well as similar games that were called, in Britain, 'camp ball', 'hurling' and 'knappan', and in continental countries, eg, 'la soule'(France), 'sollen' (The Netherlands and Belgium), and 'calcio'(Italy). As was typical of folk-games generally, these games were not highly organized. They involved 'teams' of variable and unequal sizes, and were played according to unwritten local conventions across country as well as through the streets of towns. Above all, these games were, by the more civilized standards of the present-day, rough and wild. In England in the eighteenth and nineteenth centuries, however, although they never died out completely, these games began in conjunction with the ongoing processes of state-formation and civilization, to become culturally marginalized and less popular. At the same time, they began gradually to be replaced by more formally organized and more civilized forms of football, more particularly by Association football (soccer) and Rugby football (rugger), that is, by forms that became increasingly characterized by the properties listed on the right hand side of Fig. 1. It

	Folk Football	Modern Soccer and Rugby
1.	Diffuse, informal organization implicit in the local social structure	Highly specific formal organization, institutionally differentiated at the local, regional, national and international levels
2.	Simple and unwritten customary rules, legitimated by tradition.	Formal and elaborate written rules, worked out pragmatically and legitimated by rational-bureaucratic means
3.	Fluctuating game-pattern; tendency to change through long-term and, from the viewpoint of participants, imperceptible 'drift'.	Change institutionalized through rational-bureaucratic channels.
4.	Regional variation of rules, size and shape of balls etc.	National and international standardization of rules, size and shape of balls etc.
5.	No fixed limits on territory, duration or numbers of participants.	Played on a spatially limited pitch with clearly defined boundaries, within fixed time-limits, and with a fixed number of participants, equalized between the contending sides.
6.	Strong influence of natural and social differences on the game-pattern.	Minimization, principally by means of formal rules and technological adaptations, of the influence of natural and social differences on the game-pattern: norms of equality and 'fairness'.
7.	Low role differentiation (division of labour) among the players.	High role differentiation (division of labour) among the players.
8.	Loose distinction between playing and 'spectating' roles.	Strict distinction between playing and 'spectating' roles.
9.	Low structural differentiation; several game-elements' rolled into one.	High structural differentiation; specialization around kicking, carrying and throwing, the use of sticks, etc.
10.	Informal social control by the players themselves within the context of the ongoing game.	Formal social control by officials who stand, as it were, 'outside' the game and who are appointed and certified by central legislative bodies and empowered, when a breach of rules occurs, to stop play and impose penalties graded according to the seriousness of the offence.
11.	High level of socially tolerated physical violence; emotional spontaneity; low restraint.	Low level of socially tolerated physical violence; high emotional control; high restraint.
12.	Generation in a relatively open and spontaneous form of pleasurable 'battle-excitement'.	Generation in a more controlled and 'sublimated' form of pleasurable 'battle-excitement'.
13.	Emphasis on physical force as opposed to skill.	Emphasis on skill as opposed to physical force.
14.	Strong communal pressure to participate; individual identity subordinate to group identity; test of identity in general.	Individually chosen as a recreation; Individual identity of greater importance relative to group identity; test of identity in relation to a specific skill or set of skills.
15.	Locally meaningful contests only; relative equality of playing skills among sides; no chances of national reputations or money payment.	National and international super-imposed on local contests; emergence of elite players and teams; chance to establish national and international reputations; tendency to 'monetization' of sports.

Fig. 1: The Structural Properties of Folk Football and Modern Football

is with the development of soccer as part of this latter process that I shall concern myself in this paper. Its social locus was the public schools and it occurred in conjunction with an unambiguously civilizing development of these educational establishments.

Initially formed in the Middle Ages and early modern period as charitable institutions for the education of 'poor and needy scholars and clerks' or as local grammar schools, during the eighteenth and early nineteenth centuries the British public schools were transformed into boarding establishments catering for fee-paying pupils from the middle and upper classes (2). At least two consequences followed from this transformation: (i) the class discrepancy between teachers and pupils which was inherent in the structure of a type of schools where middle class academics attempted to cater for the educational needs of boys who mostly came from higher social strata than themselves, meant that the teachers or, as they called them, 'masters', were unable to prevent the emergence of forms of self-rule by the boys; and (ii) this power and status discrepancy led to chronic indiscipline in the schools and not infrequent rebellions by the boys. Between 1728 and 1832, for example, Eton and Winchester, the two oldest public schools, each experienced at least seven rebellions, whilst Rugby, which only became a public school at the end of the eighteenth century, experienced at least four. That it is no misnomer to describe these disturbances as 'rebellions' is shown by the fact that the 1797 revolt at Rugby and the 1818 revolt at Winchester led to the Riot Act being read and could only be quelled by the militia using drawn swords and bayonets. Youthful bravado probably played a part in these rebellions. Sociologically, however, they were the most obvious surface manifestations of a long-drawn out struggle between masters and boys in which, for a long time, neither party was able to establish effective dominance over the other. The result was the gradual crystallization of a system of dual control which later came to be known as the 'prefect-fagging system'. This was a system in which the rule of masters was granted a degree of recognition in the classroom in return for the reciprocal recognition of the right of 'prefects' – the leaders among the older boys – to exercise dominance as far as extra-curricular activities were concerned.

The fagging part of the system emerged as part of the same process. The fact that the masters were unable to control the oldest boys meant that they were unable to control them in relation to their younger fellows. As a result, there emerged a dominance-hierarchy among the boys determined mainly by relativities of age and physical strength: the boys who were older and/or physically stronger 'lorded it' over those who were younger and/or physically weaker. The juniors were forced into the role of 'fags', ie, to provide menial, ego-enhancing and, in some cases, possibly also sexual services for their seniors. The strongest held sway and, as one would expect at that stage in the British civilizing process when the dominant norms of masculinity still tolerated, indeed expected, more aggressive forms of behaviour from upper and middle class males, especially of teenage boys who would not yet have formed a relatively stable adult conscience, they often exercised their power cruelly and without mercy.

The prefect-fagging system was central to the early development of football in the public schools. More particularly, at each school the game was one of the means by which the older boys asserted their dominance over juniors. One of the customary duties which developed for fags was that of 'fagging out' at football and cricket. In football, this meant they were compelled to play and restricted for the most part to the role of 'keeping goal', eg, they were ranged *en masse* along the baselines. Thus a contemporary wrote that, at Westminster in the early nineteenth century, 'the small boys, the duffers and the funk-sticks were the goalkeepers, twelve or fifteen at each end ...' 'Douling', the name given to football at Shrewsbury and reputedly derived from the Greek word for 'slave', was the same as they used for 'fagging'. And at Winchester in that period, fags, one at either end, were even used instead of goal-posts, the ball having to pass between their outstretched legs to score a goal. Fags were also used as a means of demarcating the boundaries along the sides of the pitch (2).

Just as in the folk antecedents of the modern games, football in the public schools at this stage was governed by oral rules. This meant that the ways in which boys played varied from school to school, differences deriving from the accretion over time of decisions made, eg, in relation to the geographical peculiarities of playing-areas – the game was not yet played on 'pitches' constructed and marked out for purposes of playing football – in this way leading to locally specific traditions. Despite such differences, however, handling the ball as well as kicking was allowed at *all* the schools.

All forms of public school football at this stage were also rough. In the 'scrimmages' in Charterhouse 'cloisters football', for example, 'shins would be kicked black and blue; jackets and other articles of clothing almost torn into shreds; and fags trampled under foot' (2: 56). At Westminster, 'the enemy tripped, shinned, charged with the shoulder, got you down and sat upon you - in fact, might do anything short of murder to get the ball from you' (2: 55). And in Charterhouse 'field' football, 'there were a good many broken shins, for most of the fellows had iron tips to their very strong shoes and some freely boasted of giving more than they took' (2: 56). Iron-tipped shoes were also used at Rugby where they called them 'navvies'. According to an Old Rugbeian reminiscing in the 1920s, navvies had 'a thick sole, the profile of which at the toe much resembled the ram of an ironclad', ie, a battleship (2: 55-57).

During the 1830s and 40s, at a point where the cultural marginalization of folk football was beginning to approach its peak, there began to develop in the public schools newer forms of the game, more appropriate to the social conditions, habitus, personality and values of people in an urbanizing and industrializing society in which the processes of state-formation and civilization were correlatively advancing. Centrally involved in the emergence of these newer forms were: (i) the committing of the rules to writing; (ii) a stricter demarcation and limiting of the size and shape of playing areas; (iii) the imposition of stricter limitations on the duration of matches; (iv) a reduction in the numbers taking part; (v) an equalization in the sizes of contending teams; and (vi) the introduction of stricter regulations regarding the kinds of physical force that it was legitimate to use. In a word, in this period ways of playing football characterized by the sorts of properties listed on the right hand side of Figure 1 began to emerge. It was also in the course of this process of incipient modernization that the soccer and rugby ways of playing began recognizably to emerge out of the matrix of locally differentiated public school games. Rugby appears to have been the first of these games to begin to take on its distinctive modern profile.

It is widely believed that the Rugby way of playing resulted from a deviant act by a single individual (Macrory, 1991). The individual in question was William Webb Ellis who is said in 1823 and against the then-existing rules to have picked up the ball and run with it, this deviant act hardening over time into custom. This reductionist origin myth is highly suspect (2). It is sociologically more plausible to suppose that the rugby and soccer games were, in a sense, co-produced. That is, they are best understood as having developed, not simply within particular public schools where the boys were acting in isolation, but within the wider social field formed by all the public schools at the particular stage of state-formation and civilization reached in Britain during the 1830s, 40s and 50s. It was a stage at which, largely in conjunction with urbanization and industrialization, tensions between the established, landed classes and the rising bourgeoisie were growing more intense, and, it seems reasonable to suppose, these intensifying class and status tensions were reflected in relations among the public schools, playing a part in the early development of these in many ways diametrically opposed ways of playing football.

The first public school to commit its football rules to writing was Rugby in 1845. The prefect-fagging system there had recently been reformed by Thomas Arnold, headmaster from 1828 to 1842. What Arnold basically achieved was the transformation of the Rugby variant of the prefect-fagging system from a system of dual control which was conducive to persistent disorder into a system of indirect rule which was conducive to greater harmony both in relations between staff and pupils and in those among the boys. There is, however, no evidence that Arnold was directly involved in the transformation of Rugby football which depended on this development. The rules were not committed to writing until three years after Arnold's death.

A crucial aspect of the reformed prefect-fagging system at Rugby as far as the development of football was concerned consisted of the fact that it permitted the masters to increase their power whilst simultaneously preserving a substantial measure of self-rule for the boys, especially the older boys and as far as leisure activities were concerned. A system of informal assemblies which the boys called 'levées' grew up and it was a 'Sixth Form levée' – an assembly of the senior boys – which produced the written rules of 1845. Correlation, of course, does not necessarily imply causation. However, the fact that the available evidence points towards Rugby as having been both the first public school to achieve effective reform of the prefect-fagging system and the first to commit its football rules to writing, strongly suggests that these two processes were linked.

The second public school to commit its football rules to writing seems to have been Eton, where written rules for the 'Field Game' were produced in 1847. Four among the 34 rules laid down at Eton in 1847 are of special interest for present purposes. They are as follows:

8. The goal sticks are to be seven feet out of the ground: a goal is gained when the ball is kicked between them provided it is not over the level of the top of them.
9. The space between each goal stick is to be eleven feet.
22. Hands may only be used to stop the ball, or touch it when behind. The ball must not be carried, thrown or struck by the hand.
29. A player is considered to be sneaking when only three, or less than three, of the opposite side are before him and may not kick the ball.[5]

The first three of these rules were diametrically opposite to their counterparts at Rugby where carrying and scoring by kicking the ball above H-shaped posts were legislated for in the rules of 1845. They can thus be considered as legislating for an embryonic form of soccer. So can the rule regarding 'sneaking', the evocative Eton term for 'offside'. Why should the boys at Eton have wanted to produce a game of this type, based on a taboo on the use of hands? One doubtful possibility is that the Etonians produced an entirely kicking game in isolation, completely oblivious to what was happening regarding football at other public schools. However, despite what were, by present-day standards, the relatively crude means of communication available in Britain in the mid-nineteenth century, it seems likely that the boys at the leading public schools would have had some knowledge of the core features of each others' games and that the Etonians are unlikely to have been 'cultural dopes'. They considered their school to be <u>the</u> leading public school. It was the second oldest, only Winchester being able to take pride in a longer pedigree. Having been founded by Henry VI in 1440, Eton was able to boast about being a royal foundation. Moreover, being located next to Windsor, it continued to have connections with the royal court and to recruit its pupils mainly from the highest social strata. The 1840s were a decade in which the significance of sports participation was growing in the public schools and universities, and one can easily imagine how the boys at Eton would have reacted to the development of a distinctive way of playing football at Rugby, in their eyes at the time an obscure Midlands establishment which catered primarily for parvenus.

Although founded as a grammar school in 1567, Rugby did not acquire the constitution of a public school until the 1780s, and it was only under Thomas Arnold in the 1830s that its fame began noticeably to spread and, with it, the fame of the Rugby way of playing football. As late as the 1840s, evidence suggests that Harrow boys – Harrow is the second highest status of the public schools and geographically the closest to Eton – did not yet regard Rugby as a 'full' or 'proper' public school, a feeling-state that was in all probablity more widely shared at the time. By developing a distinctive game, it seems reasonable to suppose, the Rugby boys were hoping, perhaps with the encouragement of Arnold and his staff, to draw attention to themselves as if by saying: 'Look, we're a new school and we deserve to be treated with greater respect because we've developed our own way of playing football'. Although no direct evidence about such a competitive process has yet been unearthed, it is similarly reasonable to suppose that, by developing a form of football which was equally distinctive and in key respects diametrically opposite to the game at Rugby, the Etonians were deliberately attempting to put the 'upstart' Rugbeians in their place and to 'see off' this challenge to Eton's status as *the* leading public school in *all* respects. Use of the hands, of course, is a key distinguishing feature of humans. By placing an absolute taboo on the use of these 'natural implements' in their way of playing football, the Etonians were imposing on themselves a demand for the exercise of a high degree of restraint in their play. By playing in such a way, they would have been able to demonstrate their superiority over the 'vulgar' Rugbeians whose form of football accentuated the use of hands even beyond the level permitted more generally in the football of the nineteenth century public schools.

The Eton field game, probably produced in a context of Eton-Rugby rivalry in the mid-19th century, thus seems to have been the first prototype of modern soccer. The second prototype seems to have been produced at the University of Cambridge in 1863 where the following rule was laid down: 'the ball, when in play, may be stopped by any part of the body but not be held or hit by the hands, arms or shoulders' (2). A major axis of tension in Cambridge football relations at that time was that between Old Etonian and Old Rugbeian undergraduates. For example, we hear that at Trinity College in 1848, 'the Eton men howled at the Rugby men for handling the ball' (2). They evidently regarded it as 'vulgar', a fact which is fully consistent with the hypothesis – and it is worth stressing that, until more direct evidence has been unearthed, it remains no more than a hypothesis – that Eton-Rugby tension and rivalry played a crucial part in the early bifurcation of the soccer and rugby games.

Tension between the advocates of a handling, carrying and kicking game and the advocates of a game in which the use of hands was taboo also surfaced at the inaugural meetings of the Football Association which took place towards the end of 1863. At these meetings, the Cambridge rules were used to drive out the advocates of the Rugby-way of playing, and the bifurcation of the rugby and soccer forms of football which, if my hypothesis holds water, can be traced to Eton-Rugby rivalry in the 1840s began to be consolidated on a national level. Interestingly, with aristocratic Eton giving the lead and strongly supported by other prestigious schools such as Harrow, Charterhouse and Westminster, soccer had, at this time, higher social class associations than the rugby game. Also interesting is the fact that the initial rules of the Football Association continued to allow handling in the case of a 'fair catch'. It was not until 1882 that the taboo on handling became absolute for all players except the goalkeeper.

Soccer, then, had emerged in a recognizably modern form by 1882. By that time, it had already started to spread in Britain both regionally and down the class hierarchy. It had started to spread internationally, too. The first German club was formed in Hannover in 1878, the first in the Netherlands in 1879, the first in Italy in 1890, and the first in France in 1892. FIFA was formed in 1904 with seven members and, by 1994, the number had grown to 190. By that time, soccer had become a truly 'world game'. In Britain, it had also become 'the people's game' because, as it spread down the class hierarchy, the upper and middle classes increasingly abandoned it for rugby, thus reversing the class polarities associated with these games when they first emerged,

The world-wide popularity of soccer relative to rugby and its American offshoot, can be accounted for partly in terms of the relative simplicity and hence easy understandability of its rules, and partly in terms of what Sugden and Tomlinson (16) have called its 'democratic' character, ie, the fact that its rules do not place such a premium on size and strength. The relative openness of soccer, ie, the absence of scrums, scrimmages and mauls, permits a ballet-like character to be imparted to play at the highest levels, and this helps to explain its relative success as a spectator sport. In placing less emphasis on size, strength and physical contact, it can also be said to be more 'civilized' than the rugby and American games. How, then, is the world-wide association of soccer with hooliganism to be explained? This raises complex issues but part of the answer appears to lie in two facts: firstly that soccer became, world-wide, the people's game; and secondly that, despite the existence of variations between countries lower class males everywhere in our still predominantly patriarchal world are more liable to fight openly and in public than are males from the middle and upper classes. They are also more likely to 'let themselves go' in public and to behave provocatively, thus unintentionally triggering fights (3).

Football hooliganism thus adds a de-civilizing element to the most civilized of the football games. Further pressures in this direction come on the playing side through the competitive tensions engendered by the game's global spread. However, such de-civilizing pressures only represent a disconfirmation of Elias's theory if it is wrongly read as a theory of inevitable and unilinear progress, which I established at the beginning of this paper it is not.

References

1. Dunning, E. 'On Problems of the Emotions in Sport and Leisure: Critical and Counter-Critical Comments on the Conventional and Figurational Sociologies of Sport and Leisure', *Leisure Studies,* 15, 185-207 0261-4367, pp. 185-207, 1996.
2. Dunning, E. and Sheard, K. *Barbarians, Gentlemen and Players: a Sociological Study of the Development of Rugby Football,* Oxford, Martin Robertson. 1979.
3. Dunning, E., Murphy, P. and Williams, J. *The Roots of Football Hooliganism,* London, Routledge. 1988.
4. Dunning, E., 'Sport in the Civilizing Process', in Dunning, E., Maguire, J. and Pearton, R. (eds), *The Sports Process: a Comparative and Developmental Approach, Champaign, Ill., Human Kinetics,* pp 39-70, 1993.
5. Dunning, E., *Sport Matters: Sociological Studies of Sport, Violence and Civilization,* London, Routledge. 1999.
6. Elias, N. *Über den Prozess der Zivilisation,* Basle, Haus zum Falken (2 vols). 1939.
7. Elias, N. 'Introduction' to Elias, N. and Dunning, E. *Quest for Excitement: Sport and Leisure in the Civilizing Process,* Oxford, Blackwell. 1986.
8. Elias, N. *The Symbol Theory,* London, Sage. 1991.
9. Elias, N. *The Civilizing Process,* (integrated single volume edition), Oxford, Blackwell. 1994.
10. Elias, N. *The Germans: Power Struggles and the Development of Habitus in the Nineteenth and Twentieth Centuries,* Cambridge, Polity. 1996.

11. Elias, N. and Dunning, E. *Quest for Excitement: Sport and Leisure in the Civilizing Process*. Oxford, Blackwell. 1986.

12. Giddens, A. *The Constitution of Society,* Cambridge, Polity. 1984.

13. Horne, J. and Jary, D. 'The Figurational Sociology of Sport of Elias and Dunning: an Exposition and Critique', in Horne, J., Jary, D. and Tomlinson, A. (eds), *Sport, Leisure and Social Relations,* London, Routledge. 1987.

14. Krüger, M. *Körperkultur and Nationsbildung: die Geschichte des Turnens in der Reichsgründungsära,* Schorndorf, Karl Hofmann. 1996.

15. Mangan, J. A. *Athleticism in the Victorian and Edwardian Public School,* Cambridge, Cambridge University Press. 1981.

16. Sugden, J. and Tomlinson, A. *FIFA and the Struggle for World Football,* Cambridge, Polity. 1998.

17. Williams, R. *Keywords: a Vocabulary of Culture and Society,* London, Fontana. 1976.

Footnotes

1   Use of time-reference terms such as 'modern' and 'post-modern' is liable to be confusing, especially in a period of rapid global change such as we are currently experiencing. It is liable, for example, to be conducive to endless and fruitless debates about the borderlines between these so-called eras and to the use of a potentially endless series of moderators as in, eg, 'post-post-modern', 'post-post-post modern' etc.

2   The concept of habitus has been popularized in recent years by Pierre Bourdieu. (See his Distinction: a Social Critique of the Judgement of Taste, Trans. Richard Nice, London, Routledge and Kegan Paul, 1979). However, it was a term commonly used in German sociology between the two World Wars and first appears on pxi of the Preface to the 1939 edition of Elias's Über den Prozess der Zivilisation. In Elias's usage, the concept means 'second nature' or 'embodied social learning'.

3   See, e.g. the discussion of Elias by Giddens (12) and Horne and Jary (13).

4   The term 'public school' refers in Britain to boarding schools which cater primarily for the offspring of the upper and middle classes. The British equivalent to 'public school' in its literal or American sense is 'state school'. For an insightful and scholarly study of of sports and games in the nineteenth century British public Schools, see 15.

5   A copy of the 1847 Eton rules was unearthed by Graham Curry, a Leicester postgraduate student, when he was researching in the archives at Eton.

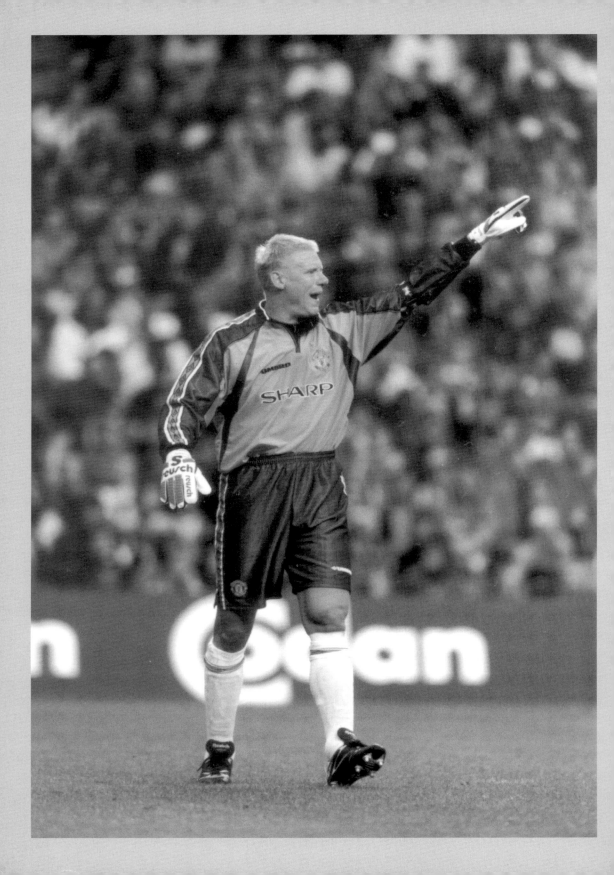

'No Boundaries to Ambition'
Soccer labour migration and the case of Nordic/Scandinavian players in England

David Stead & Joseph Maguire

Synopsis

This chapter focuses on the growth and complexity of international sport labour migration. Attention is drawn to the significance of the phenomenon in soccer and explanations for this are offered. A case study of the movement of Nordic/Scandinavian players into English professional soccer provides insights into the development of a particular soccer migration route and the characteristics and experiences of the players who have travelled along it. The frequency and form of this migration is mapped out from season 1946/1947 to season 1996/1997. Interview and questionnaire data provide insights into the migrant's motivation and objectives, migration preparation and choice of England as a destination. The personal and professional challenges faced by migrants are examined.

Introduction

An increasingly important feature of global commercial activity has been the rise of the internationally mobile professional. The world of sport, including soccer, has not been immune from such developments. The incidence and impact of skilled labour migration have become highly significant factors in the analysis of modern sport. A growing number of elite professional, primarily male, athletes from many sports are now selling their labour outside their home countries. Sports affected include both rugby codes (6, 23), basketball (10, 20), baseball (8), ice hockey (4, 16), cricket (7, 18), track and field (1) and American Football (11). However, as Bale and Maguire (2 p.2) have suggested, the sports labour migration process is "arguably most pronounced in soccer" (3, 9, 19).

We have examined this sport based migration in the context of investigations into sport and processes of globalization (11, 12, 13, 14, 15, 16, 17, 18, 19). Several of the key issues involved have been addressed, a conceptual model proposed and a research agenda outlined (2, 15). Various empirically based case studies have undertaken, one of which is the central concern of this paper.

Our soccer migration research has concentrated on three interrelated areas. We have mapped out the broad patterns and structures that characterise the movement of players within Europe, and within and between various regions of the globe (19). In addition, we have explored the meaning and experience of labour migration for the migrant players themselves. A further line of enquiry has been to consider of the significance of labour migration as part of the political economy, firstly, of soccer and secondly, of global sport more broadly (5, 21, 22). The study of Nordic/Scandinavian players in English soccer discussed in this chapter represents an example of how we have combined our mapping work with enquiries into the lived experiences of migrant players. This latter concern has involved the examination of the characteristics of the players, their migration motives, objectives and preparation and the personal and professional challenges they face.

We have offered some tentative explanations for the patterning of global, but more specifically European soccer migration (19). In doing this, we have paid due regard to the global political economy of soccer and to the various key organisations or sectors involved and the power balance and tensions that exist between them. Attention has been drawn to a wide range of relevant political, economic and cultural processes and how they interweave to structure the recruitment and retention of players. The kinds of soccer related processes identified include:
- the ascribing of status to particular leagues or playing characteristics to certain nationalities,
- the political, economic and playing success ambitions of particular clubs, leagues and national associations,
- the development and exploitation of new talent sources,

- the spectator's acceptance of, indeed demand for, cosmopolitan teams.

Relevant processes of a wider non soccer specific kind have also been highlighted and they include:
- the ongoing impact of colonial heritages and cultural linkages and non sport related migration experience,
- cultural and legal encouragement or discouragement of migration,
- economic dependency and exploitation,
- political change e.g. in Eastern Europe and greater political interdependency e.g. the moves towards European integration.

The various groups involved in the international movement of players usually interact within prescribed boundaries and conventions and with little difficulty and controversy. However, in recent times, soccer migration has become a high profile topic. More players are moving internationally. New talent sources like the Eastern European countries have come to the fore. Clubs in such countries as England are now recruiting significant numbers of players from abroad. The costs and benefits of these developments can be the subject of considerable debate. One factor has been the emergence of players' agents. They have appeared in ever increasing numbers and are vigorously selling their clients on the international transfer market. The Federation Internationale de Football Association (FIFA), soccer's world governing body, has reacted to concerns about the activities of these agents and has established a licensing scheme in order to exercise some quality control over them.

Another, and major, development has been the Bosman case. This successful legal challenge by the Belgian player, Jean Marc Bosman, to labour mobility restrictions placed on him has led to greater freedoms for athletes within the European Union countries. It has also resulted in the abolition of the foreign player quotas in European soccer leagues and competitions that were a disincentive on clubs to recruit internationally. The full impact of the Bosman case on soccer is yet to be established. Will it lead to a greater disparity of playing standards in and between the European leagues as the economically rich clubs monopolise the best talent? Given that the more powerful clubs can recruit foreign players as they wish, will this lead to the underdevelopment of future talent and the lack of employment opportunities for existing indigenous players? What will be the impact on the size of transfer fees and the length of player contracts? Our best estimate is that elite clubs from core European soccer economies e.g. the leagues in England, Italy and Spain will become more powerful following the Bosman ruling. Although some of these elite clubs have retained youth development programmes, the pressure for instant success will persuade them to buy extensively from abroad. One outcome of Bosman may be to place more emphasis on the interests of the players themselves. To a degree, they are now in a better position to exercise greater control over their careers, including the international transfer option. The following case study is therefore timely in that migrant player motives and objectives are addressed. It is a study that provides some revealing insights into the sport migration phenomenon and the world of elite professional soccer.

Case study: Nordic/Scandinavian players in elite English soccer

The history and extent of the Nordic/Scandinavian presence

Many factors lie behind the coming of the 'foreign legions' of soccer players into England. Some relate to changes in the English game whilst others are of wider origin. The prices of players in the English domestic market place have risen considerably. A large scale injection of TV money has increased the spending power of the top English clubs. The aforementioned Bosman rulings and subsequent changes in soccer's regulations have had an impact. More players have turned to England in pursuit of the full time professional career denied to them by the economic situation of soccer in their homelands. The English clubs have taken advantage of the new talent pipelines that have emerged or opened up, not just in Europe but in such areas as North America and Australia.

Much of the media coverage of the changing nature of the English soccer workforce has centred on the questions, indeed risks, faced by the purchasers of the foreign talent. But what of the players themselves?

To what degree is their movement a leap into the unknown? What challenges do they face and with what outcomes?

In order to address such questions we chose to focus on those Nordic/ Scandinavian players who had appeared in English soccer. The levels of English soccer participation of male elite players from Denmark, Finland, Iceland, Norway and Sweden were established for each season from 1946/1947 until 1996/1997. Approaches were made to those players who were in England in 1996/1997 and to former migrants. Twenty seven players responded by the completion of questionnaires and/or by giving interviews. In order to respect confidentiality, pseudonyms are used when specific interview data is referred to later in this chapter. The Nordic/Scandinavian players were selected for our enquiries because of their prominence amongst the migrants in England. Their high level of education and competency in the English language were also important concerns. They represented a group of players who would be most likely to respond favourably to a research enquiry. We were aware that such helpful factors about these players would lead to difficulties in making any definitive conclusions about other nationalities. Ironically, problems were encountered in obtaining responses to both the interview and questionnaire requests. The players' unwillingness to respond can be explained by such factors as apathy, fear of what can be controversial subject matter or, possibly, concern about language competence in an interview situation. These elite professional players also get inundated by approaches for interviews etc, including many from their home countries. They tend to be wary of media requests and may not differentiate between these enquiries and those from academics. The players' reaction to our specific approaches may have also owed something to a rather sensitive context. During the life of the research project, investigations into the financial transactions involved in Nordic/Scandinavian player transfers to England were instigated by soccer governing bodies and the police.

English soccer has always been characterised by the inclusion of large numbers of players from the other parts of the United Kingdom and from Ireland. Players from other countries have appeared but it is only in the 1990s that the English game has taken on the highly cosmopolitan look that it has today (Fig. 1). In season 1994/1995, excluding other UK and Irish citizens, some 59 players from 22 countries were playing in the Premier League, England's top league. Forty of these were Europeans from 13 different countries. Two seasons later the number of migrants had risen to 109 players from 32 countries with the presence of Europeans increasing to 88 players from 20 countries. This level of involvement is out of a total Premier League workforce of approximately 500 players. Significantly, 17 of the European players in 1994/95, i.e. 42.5%, were from Nordic/Scandinavian countries. By 1996/1997, their numbers had increased to 28 players. This, however, represented a reduction to 31.8% of all the Europeans in the league. English clubs' recruitment strategies have become more diverse. Nevertheless, the Nordic/Scandinavian players remain the largest bloc of European imports.

Our detailed mapping of the presence of Nordic/Scandinavian players has extended beyond just the elite division. Increasingly, the Premier League data only reveal part of the migration into England.

	Season			
	1991/1992	1994/1995	1995/1996	1996/1997
Number of Foreign Players	37	59	77	109
Number of Donor Countries	18	22	30	32
Number of European Players	29	40	54	88
Number of European Donors	13	13	19	20
*Excludes players from the other UK countries and Ireland				
Sources: European Football Yearbooks/'Playfair' Football Who's Who				

Fig. 1 Foreign Players in the Top Division of English League Soccer

Detailed examination of all levels of English professional soccer in a fifty season period until 1995/1996 has enabled us to trace the expansion of the migration route (Fig. 2). From the 1946/1947 season until the late 1970s, players from the Nordic/Scandinavian countries did appear in England but never more than 3 in any one season. The 15 years up to 1995/1996 saw a more regular presence with a steep climb in the numbers of migrants. In 1989/1990 there were 14 players involved and six seasons later this total had reached 36. A total of 80 different players came to England in the fifty years examined. The fact that 36 of them played in the 1995/1996 season again emphasises the

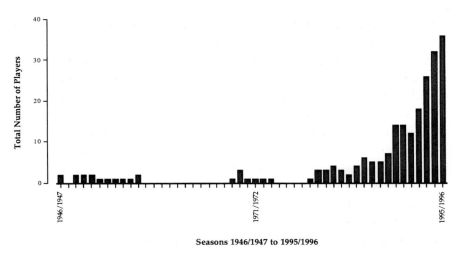

Fig. 2 The Presence of Nordic/Scandinavian Players in English League Soccer

significance of recent developments. Indeed, a review of data from the 1996/1997 season revealed that no less than 51 Nordic/Scandinavian players had taken part in at least one English league match during that season.

The 80 players involved in the specific 50 year period came from the five donor countries as follows: Denmark 33%, Finland 8%, Iceland 8%, Norway 32% and Sweden 19% (Fig. 3). Denmark provided 27 of these players. Up to 1984/1985, there was never more than 2 Danes present in any one season but in 1995/1996 there were nine. An

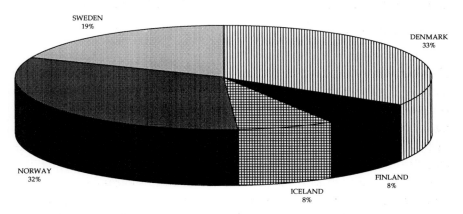

Fig. 3 The Sources of Nordic/Scandinavian Soccer Players in England 1946/1947 to 1995/1996

occasional Finnish citizen has played, with 6 in total having been involved, two of whom participated in 1995/1996. Whilst one Icelander amateur played briefly in 1946/1947, it was not until 1984/1985 that one of his countrymen appeared again. There have only been 6 Icelanders in total with 3 having played in England in 1995/1996. Twenty six Norwegians have played in the fifty seasons. Whilst this is a figure similar to the Danish total, the recent increase in their presence is far more dramatic. Until 1989/1990 there had only once been as many as two players present in a season. By 1995/1996 a total of sixteen Norwegians were playing for English clubs. The 1989/1990 season was also notable for the presence of 3 Swedish players. There had been almost no previous involvement. By 1995/1996, the number of Swedes had risen to six.

The characteristics of the Nordic/Scandinavian imports

How do these Nordic/Scandinavian imports compare with the other foreign players in England? A number of key characteristics have been examined for a sample season 1996/1997. These have included age, number of seasons in England and other international movement history, international representative experience and transfer fee on entering English soccer. The ages of all the 213 foreign players in England during 1996/1997 were established using the first of January 1997 as the census day. The average age of these players was 26.32 years. The Nordic/Scandinavian players' average was almost the same at 26.37 years. Interestingly, one English manager, David Pleat, now with Tottenham Hotspur, has said that "the mid twenties is the right vintage for the imported player". Most of the foreign imports were new to the English game with 65.3% of them being in only their first or second season. This was the case with the Nordic/Scandinavian players. Eleven of the 15 Danes were in their first year. Nearly 50% of the Norwegians were in a similar situation as were 70% of the Swedes. Some of the players in England had arrived having had other international soccer migration experience. At least a quarter of the Nordic/Scandinavian players had played outside their home countries prior to coming to England.

What is the calibre of the foreign players? One yardstick is evidence of international representative experience. In 1996/1997, 63.6% of all the foreign players in England were full internationals. The equivalent figure for Nordic/Scandinavian players was almost 70%. As many as 15, i.e. 75%, of the Norwegians had played at this level. Nine out of the 15 Danes were similarly qualified. An alternative method of assessing the standards and, indeed, of establishing market trends and nationality differences, is to examine the range of transfer fees paid. For example, the 26 Eastern European and 8 Italian imports in to England cost an average of £1,285,385 and £3.980,000 per player respectively. The other end of the transfer scale included players from such countries as Australia and the USA. Some of these had arrived on 'free' transfers. This had happened with ten out the 23 Australians. Enquiries with the Nordic/Scandinavian players suggest that they see themselves as relatively inexpensive, a characteristic making them particularly attractive to English clubs. They believe they are looked upon as 'good value', especially when compared with the Eastern Europeans, Italians and South Americans. The data on Nordic/Scandinavian players in England in 1996/1997 suggests that they do not command the highest level of transfer fees. The average fee was £708,435. However, this is not to say that there are no multi-million pound transfers involving Nordic/Scandinavian players or that there are no differences between the five nationalities concerned.

In general, the Nordic/Scandinavian players were not untypical of the foreign imports as a group. They tended to be fairly mature in terms of age if not in English soccer experience. They were high quality as assessed by international representative qualifications but somewhat average when related to the level of transfer fees they commanded. Some differences between the five nationalities were evident. The mapping out of a particular transfer route and examination of the characteristics of the players involved has helped provide a context to the examination of the actual sport migration experience.

Migrant player experiences and views

Migration motives, objectives and preparation

Whilst many factors influenced the decision to play abroad, a consistent theme from the interviews conducted was the centrality of a highly personal quest for greater soccer experience. This emphasis is evident from a Norwegian player (Arild) who, when asked why he moved, said: "firstly for myself, to come and play here, second, the higher salary and, third, to get a language". The principal motivation for migrating appears to centre on the opportunity of experiencing a full-time professional career and the level of mental and physical commitment that this involves. Some 60% of questionnaire respondents rated this factor as very important. Arild commented on the significance of becoming a full time player in the following way: "hopefully you can develop everything about yourself and your skills, so its better".

The players did consider a commitment to professionalism i.e. a discipline to the way they approached their sporting life, was a strong characteristic of the Nordic/Scandinavian player. Nevertheless, another Norwegian (Vegard), observed that "in Norway they don't really call you a professional until you have played outside Norway". For many, moving abroad appeared a logical progression, a 'rite de passage'.

Clearly, a lack of full-time professional employment opportunities was a push factor. However, the players were also pulled by a strong desire to test themselves at a high level on a regular and consistent basis. A 20 year old Norwegian player (Henrik) commented that he had come "to try something new, something different from what we have in Norway, to play in a tougher league, a challenge". Not surprisingly, therefore, nearly all the Nordic/Scandinavian players rated the development of soccer skills and knowledge as an important or very important migration objective.

Skill development ambitions ranked about the same as the desire for a high salary level. The latter incentive appeared to be more about ensuring financial security rather than an interest in immediate wealth and a lifestyle to match. Although financial rewards appeared of secondary importance in questionnaire responses, the interviewed players did refer to the topic frequently. Some pointed out that the Nordic/Scandinavian players were not amongst the highest paid imports in to

England. However, others did emphasise that they were much better off financially than at home. Danish and Swedish players made specific reference to the high taxation rates back in their own countries.

England was seen as a desirable destination. The specific emphasis was placed on the attractiveness of the soccer situation. The reputation and status of the English game and the type of soccer played were seen consistently as being more important than any wider benefits of being in England. Reflecting on why he came to England, Arild pointed out that "Everyone (in Norway) knows about English football. We have seen the atmosphere every Saturday afternoon. You have the dream to play in that league". Players tended to have had little specific knowledge about the English club and area to which they moved. It was normally a matter of taking things on trust and having a certain confidence that they would be able to handle whatever they encountered. The salary and employment conditions offered by the club were the main considerations. Over 75% of the players ranked these conditions as important or very important in choosing the club. The club's status was seen as slightly less of consideration. However, a Dane (Torben) advocated joining a small club because his "chances were better to play every time than at a big club". To be a migrant and out of the first team can be particularly stressful. One young Swedish player (Magnus) was not being selected. He complained: "I haven't had a fair chance to show how good I am".

Less than 25% of the questionnaire respondents considered that the particular city and region in which their English club was situated had been of importance. There were players who spoke of the benefits of being in a big city. One young and single Norwegian (Vegard) offered the advice "move close to London or you better have a family if you move North". The players' knowledge of English soccer and their enthusiasm for it, had been developed primarily through the media in their home countries. Over 60% of the players cited the TV coverage of the English games as very important. Many reflected on how this exposure had been instrumental in fuelling ambitions to be internationally mobile.

The majority of players had represented their country and it was clear that an important sharing of information about England occurred when they met up for international matches or squad training sessions. Ten, i.e. 55%, of the Nordic/Scandinavian respondents who played in the 1996/1997 season referred to advice from former migrants to England. Nearly 75% of the players noted the relevance of having played against English opposition. This happened while playing for their country at various levels and/or for their clubs in European club competitions. It is also not uncommon for English teams to undertake preseason tours to the Nordic/Scandinavian countries.

The players' wider knowledge base about England and the English way of life had come mainly from school, college and the media. Some players emphasised the international awareness of the Nordic/Scandinavian peoples. For example, one player (Mikael) pointed out: "England was not so strange. First of all people in Sweden are very educated about other countries. We read a lot about outside".

Around 50% of the players reported that they had been very well prepared for the move. Only one considered that his preparations had not been sufficient. The interviewees reflected frequently on their psychological readiness to become sports migrants. Confidence was the key for some players. As a Dane (Jens) put it: "My self confidence was at a very high level so I felt I can go there because I knew it was a big club, big city so I needed all the confidence in myself I could get together".

The players were keen to offer advice to potential migrants. The emphasis was on the need to have the right mental approach. Another Danish player (Morten) suggested that they "look in the mirror, see if they are ready or not, and make sure they are not lying to themselves because if they do they will not have success over here and therefore always think about going home again". The need to be open minded was recommended frequently, as was the value of having a good level of maturity as a player. Clear about objectives, prepared for the move and fairly informed but generally open minded about England, the players had then to face the challenge of being a migrant in a foreign land.

Living as a Foreign Sportsman in England

In general, the Nordic/Scandinavian soccer migrants appear to be adept at dealing with both the personal and professional changes arising from migration. We will first consider the wider personal side of this experience. Our earlier study of cricketers highlighted the difficulties sports migrants can face being away from relations and friends. Loneliness was not an uncommon experience (18). When asked about the personal issues they may have faced in England, the soccer players placed overwhelming importance on maintaining relationships with people back home. Like the cricketers, the telephone was often seen as a vital and much used lifeline. One Norwegian player (Carsten) spoke of "big phone bills, massive phone bills".

Some experience of loneliness was reported. Over 25% of the players stated that it had been a frequent issue for them. Around 60% of the remaining players also reported the experience, although it had been infrequent. The concern appeared more prevalent with the younger and/or unaccompanied player. The experience may not be confined to the first few weeks. It could also occur when the excitement of the move had died down. Soccer is an unpredictable and demanding career. You can be injured or lose form and you are then out of the team. The objectives of the international move may not be being met. Some of the interviewed players referred to having experienced such difficulties. Living far away from home can heighten the impact. One Icelandic player (Thordur) commented on the time when his initial period of success had come to an end. He said: "it was like hitting a wall, all of a sudden you had a bad game, the press is on my back, I am tired physically and mentally and there is no one to help you".

Some players spoke of this vulnerability and underlined the benefits of having family or friends living with them. Most of those interviewed had been accompanied by a wife or girlfriend. One player (Jens) said of the arrival of his girlfriend: "It helped me tremendously. Once she was over here I really had someone to talk to about a lot of things, practical things. There is high pressure when you play at a big club. To be able to go home and speak about that and to get rid of some of the pressure was very important".

Some players were in long term relationships and had children, whilst, for others, the move away from their homeland involved a new and potentially stressful phase in what may have been a relatively new relationship. Jens, whose relationship with his girlfriend eventually broke down said: "she should have had a job and maybe it would have worked out. She was at home every day all the time. Once I got back from training she would want entertainment and I would want rest". We do believe there are specific questions to be asked about the situation of these 'migrants by association'. For example, to what degree do they experience loneliness?

Competency in the host country's language was often referred to as an important factor in a successful move abroad for players and their partners. As many as 60% of the questionnaire respondents rated this issue as very important. Most of the players arrived with a good command of English but recognised the need to develop this as quick as possible.

Overseas cricketers developed and used a supportive network based on their fellow countrymen playing in England (18). The soccer players also mentioned these kinds of networks although they appear more informal and less significant. Only 25% of the players rated such links as important to their personal support. However, there were references to supportive grouping of Nordic/Scandinavian, and, indeed, other foreign players, at particular clubs. Whilst the establishment of this kind of enclave may have been helpful to the players concerned, it could be potentially divisive by separating the migrants from the indigenous players. Although he played the incident down, one player (Jens) spoke of how a conversation in 'Scandinavian' with a fellow migrant had been met "by a lot of foul language" from his team mates and the demand "don't talk that language, just speak English while you are here". As it is, whilst the players tended to be positive towards their English team mates and the reception they had received, few saw them as an important source of personal support. A Finnish player (Petri) enjoyed the openness of the English players and had found them easy to get on with. However, he did point out that "you always end up being the foreigner".

Assistance was forthcoming from officials of employing clubs, particularly when the player arrived. However, some players felt that this kind of personal support should have been available longer. For some, there was a feeling that clubs are concerned when the signing is news but fail to appreciate that the migrants players problems can persist, or indeed develop, once the excitement has died down. One player (Magnus) remarked: "they help a little at first but then you are just a player like everyone else ... they expect this guy is a good player ... we've paid all this money ... we don't have to worry about him, his personal life ... he can deal with that himself". Some players were full of praise for their clubs. Jens mentioned a manager who had been a migrant player and said: "what he did, his actions showed me that he understood that he had experienced some of the problems I do". When clubs were seen as supportive so the players expressed a wish to reciprocate. As

Torben put it: "if you are happy with the club you also want to do something when you are playing".

Agents sometimes played a significant part in not only the contractual side of the move but also by acting as a friend and adviser on more personal issues. Generally, the role of agents was seen as positive but there was some evidence of apprehension. As (Mikael) remarked: "the thing is if you don't know them personally, if they can have a profit in you, you don't really know if they are good or bad until afterwards". However, one of the Danish players (Jens) was more philosophical and said: "If I did not have an agent I wouldn't be here. What he gets out of it is not a problem. If I get what I want. If I have done well. It doesn't matter if he makes a million".

The English Soccer Experience

As with the challenge of personal changes, the players appear to cope well with their new soccer surroundings. This is not to say that no significant difficulties were encountered. In general, the players' response was to accept the situation and to adjust accordingly. There are problems coming to terms with the more hierarchical forms of management in England and with the different coaching styles and training timetables. Over half the players rated dealing with managers and coaches, and their coaching styles, as important employment issues. The players tended to find the English managers to be more distant than those back home. A Finn (Petri) said: "We are used to talking to the manager and saying what we think". Reflecting on his English experience, he commented that "sometimes the manager being a bit further away is a good thing, sometimes its a negative thing. It's a bit like I experienced in the Army". A difference in the way the English professional responded to managers was identified. In general, they were perceived to be far more deferential. There was the acknowledgement of distinct status differences in English professional soccer.

Despite the more distant managerial approach, some players found the actual coaching styles to be more informal and less scientific than they had experienced. Difficulties were encountered in adapting to this change. Reference was made to receiving less individual attention. A Norwegian (Carsten) commented: "The training wasn't really structured. You train to train. We didn't train to get better. It was really frustrating". For some players, full-time did not mean anything more than they had experienced back home. Pontus Kaamark, a Swedish player formerly at Leicester City, has been quick to "dispel the myths" of the part-time nature of the Nordic/Scandinavian soccer. He has been quoted as saying: "That is utter rubbish. Yes, we do have other jobs but we still train every day ... football still comes very much first" (Foxes Magazine October 1996 p. 31). The players did tend to find the English training regimes to be less time consuming. A difficult contradiction for them was the intensity of games and the non intensity of training. They had come to realise that the emphasis is on recovery training as a response to pressure of the matches. However, it was not easy to adjust. As one Dane (Jens) put it: "in the beginning I wanted to train harder. I felt I'd lost my sharpness."

The amount of free time was sometimes a problem. One player (Carsten) said: "its so much relaxed but too much time for my liking". A Dane (Torben) advised that you should: "make sure you have family and friends so you can do something with your free time because there is a lot of it in English football". The lighter training regimes were seen as a bonus for players with children. One (Arild) remarked: "I think the perfect way to raise children is to be a professional footballer". Whilst the training commitment may not have been time consuming, players referred frequently to the importance of being prepared to work hard. Most players reported difficulties coming to terms with the large number of matches they were expected to play in English soccer. Nearly 30% of them saw this as an very important issue and most of the rest considered it important. It was not just a physical thing, for as a Norwegian (Carsten) commented, it is "very hard, very hard on your head playing that many games".

The playing styles were generally seen as similar which was a factor helping players to adapt quickly. However, nearly 60% of the players rated playing styles as an important issue. The speed and physicality of the English game had been a problem for some players. As one (Petri) said: "the emphasis is on being strong, winning the battle". Most players said that had realised that this was going to be the case but the early days were hard.

Coaches, fans and others had high expectations of the imported cricketers and this was often felt as a heavy burden by the players concerned. (18). Such pressure was not so evident amongst the Nordic/Scandinavian soccer players in this study. However, they do not represent the most high profile or best paid imports in to England and therefore the expectations on them may be more qualified than it is for other soccer migrants. The status of the indigenous professional is also a factor. As Mikael commented: "it takes away the pressure a little bit because they (the English) know that their own stars in football are stars all over the world".

The English soccer player may well be feeling threatened by the foreign players. Livelihoods and career prospects may be seen to be at risk. Such factors could have caused difficulties for the Nordic/Scandinavian players in dealing with their indigenous colleagues. However, they considered themselves well accepted. Nearly 60% of the players rated developing relationships with team-mates as an important issue. Jens did feel the indigenous player was resigned to the presence of the imports and said: "the English player accepts that they are not bigger than the club, they are there for the club, so if the club wants them, then the foreigners will be there". Many players felt that their ability and dedication were central to them earning the respect and acceptance of their indigenous colleagues. However, one player (Jens) only really broke the ice after playing the piano. He remarked: "I felt I had contributed with something because I couldn't crack jokes in English, I couldn't tell all those long stories. It was impossible for me".

The migrants respected the indigenous players even though they recognised differences in commitment and soccer culture. A Finn (Petri) saw merit in the way: "English players just get on with the job and don't stop to think of unnecessary things and that way they handle everything". However, a Norwegian (Arild) was less positive. He said: "the English professional knows nothing else apart from being a pro. He acts like other players. They come in do what the coaches tell them to do. They go back home and do nothing". For some of the migrants there were indeed aspects of English soccer culture that were seen as alien and unattractive. The response was one of accommodation rather than assimilation. Definitions of professionalism came to the fore. Kaamark, created some anger when he was reported as criticising his English team-mates for their level of alcohol consumption. The player strongly denied the report and apologised to his colleagues but the incident was suggestive of a different soccer culture (Leicester Mercury 21st February 1997 p. 56). Some of the interviewees did draw attention to the question of drinking. They were not always criticising their colleagues but rather pointing to a different culture, one they had little interest in joining.

When asked about why English clubs are keen to employ Nordics/Scandinavians, the players emphasised the disciplined approach in their work and a high level of adaptability. A willingness to work hard was another characteristic mentioned and one that several players saw as vital for anyone considering a move to England. One player (Mikael) said: "it's some kind of security for the club if they buy a Swedish player. They know he is going to try and do his best". A Dane (Torben) commented: "we are easy to work with. I think because of how we are brought up in our country". The players also spoke of their value in comparison with other nationals. A Norwegian (Arild) remarked: "they know we are not used to luxury as maybe players from other countries". The players' own assessment of themselves was echoed by the English journalist, Neil Harman, who, in reference to Norwegian imports, wrote: "Almost without exception, they are the uncomplaining, honest, dedicated face of foreign football" (Daily Mail, 9th December 1996 p.60). The Norwegian player, Stig Inge Bjornebye, has spoken in a similar vein: "An English manager knows what he is getting with a Norwegian player. He is not getting any problems he doesn't need, in other words, he is getting a sportsman who respects himself and those around him" (The Observer – Sport, 27th October 1996 p.5).

Interestingly, nearly all the respondents rated their technical skill levels as less important to employers. This may be some modesty but it does reflect the self improvement motivation of this particular group of athletes. Whilst the players focused on the personal characteristics of the Nordic/Scandinavian imports, many also recognised soccer's political economy at work. They recognised their position in the market place. There was an acknowledgement that the Nordic/Scandinavian player has tended to be a low cost option for English clubs as compared with the likes of the Brazilians and Italians and, indeed, the indigenous professional. Away from just the soccer context, the players pointed to their aptitude for settling quickly and easily in to new social situations. Nordic/Scandinavian players appear to have caused few problems for their English employers. A Danish player (Jens) suggested that "you don't get a lot of scandals from the Scandinavian player".

The players recognised that they were part of a larger migration revolution in English soccer. From their perspective, they tended to see that the strongest motive behind this importation of foreign labour was the desire of English clubs to improve their playing standards. They believed migrant players were being well received in England, particularly by the English fans. However, Jens explained how this support had to be earned. As he said: "from the first game you play you have to be showing the supporters that you want to work for them". The relative anonymity of the Nordic/Scandinavian player also helped in getting the fans on their side. As Jens said: "If you come from Italy you have got to deliver. Its the money. The supporters read what money you are on. You don't read what we earn. The supporters see we are not on huge wages".

Reflections

The Nordic/Scandinavian migrant players have been in the forefront of the changing composition of the English soccer workforce and, although they are now having to compete with prospective migrants from many more countries, their numbers continue to rise. Their presence may develop still further. English clubs are becoming more experienced in seeking out and employing players from the region. There are now many more England based role models for potential migrants back in the Nordic/Scandinavian countries. However, there are a wide range of supply and demand factors that will structure how the form and extent of the particular migration route will develop. Will the Nordic/Scandinavian soccer authorities seek to protect the quality of their own leagues by taking steps to encourage players to stay at home? Will proposed youth development initiatives in England lead to a more productive indigenous talent pipeline? The processes involved that lead up to a migration experience are complex. The objectives of players, and whether they continue to be met, are but one of the key concerns.

In our tentative analysis of global soccer migration patterns we have offered a number of explanations for the prevalence of the Nordic/Scandinavian players (19). We pointed to the lack of professional opportunities, financial rewards and consistently high level competition in their home countries. Whilst some club sides such as Malmö and Göteborg, (Sweden) and Brondby, (Denmark) have been successful in European competitions, there is not the financial infrastructure or the continuity of participation in high-level competition in Sweden and Denmark to persuade ambitious players to remain in the domestic leagues. We have also suggested that soccer cultures foster and promote attitudes towards certain nationalities. National stereotyping exists within the world of soccer. The personal and professional characteristics ascribed to Nordic/Scandinavian players make them attractive to foreign clubs. These qualities include high educational standards, language competencies and an aptitude for settling into new surroundings and cultures. The findings of study outlined in this chapter have both confirmed these kinds of hypotheses and extended our understanding considerably.

The particular case study we have presented reflects only one regional grouping of migrants and one host country. However, avenues of enquiry have been highlighted and the findings have been revealing. They have helped explain and emphasise the importance of international soccer migration in soccer. It is an importance that will be enhanced by the Bosman case and the far reaching interest that this has created. It is to be hoped that further studies into soccer migration will be undertaken and that these will pay due regard to impact of Bosman.

References

1. Bale, J. & Sang, J. *Kenyan running: movement culture, geography and global change.* 1996.
2. Bale, J. & Maguire, J. (eds). *The Global Sports Arena: Athletic Talent Migration in an Interdependent World.* 1994.
3. Duke, V. 'The flood from the East? Perestroika and the Migration of Sports talent from eastern Europe'. In: Bale, J. & Maguire, J. (eds). *The Global Sports Arena: Athletic Talent Migration in an Interdependent World.* pp 153-170, 1994.
4. Genest, S. 'Skating on thin ice? The international migration of Canadian ice hockey players'. In: Bale, J. & Maguire, J. (eds). *The Global Sports Arena: Athletic Talent Migration in an Interdependent World,* pp 112 -125, 1994.
5. Giulianotti, R. & Williams, J. (eds) *Game without frontiers. Football, identity and modernity,* 1994.
6. Hadfield, D. *Playing Away – Australians in British Rugby League,* 1992.
7. Hill, J. 'Cricket and the Imperial Connection: overseas players in Lancashire in the inter – war years'. In: Bale, J. & Maguire, J. (eds). *The Global Sports Arena: Athletic Talent Migration in an Interdependent World.* pp 49-62, 1994.
8. Klein, A. M. *Sugarball. The American game, the Dominican dream.* 1991.

9. Lanfranchi, P. 'The Migration of Footballers: the case of France'. In: Bale, J. & Maguire, J. (eds). *The Global Sports Arena: Athletic Talent Migration in an Interdependent World.* pp 63-77, 1994.

10. Maguire, J. 'The Commercialization of English Elite Basketball: 1972-1988'. *International Review for the Sociology of Sport* 23, 305-324, 1988.

11. Maguire, J. 'More than a Sporting "Touchdown": the Making of American Football in Britain 1982-1989'. *Sociology of Sport Journal* 7, 213-237, 1990.

12. Maguire, J. 'Hired Corporate Guns? Elite Sport Migrants in the Global Arena'. *Vrijetijd En Samenleving* 10, 19-30, 1993.

13. Maguire, J. 'Globalization, Sport and National Identities: the Empires Strike Back?'. *Society and Leisure* 16, 293-323, 1993.

14. Maguire, J. Preliminary Observations on Globalisation and the Migration of Sport Labour. *Sociological Review* 3, 452-480, 1994.

15. Maguire, J. Sport, Identity Politics and Globalization in *Sociology of Sport Journal* 11, 398-427, 1994.

16. Maguire, J. Blade Runners: Canadian Migrants, Ice Hockey and the Global Sports Process. *Journal of Sport and Social Issues* 20, 335-360, (1996).

17. Maguire, J. *Global sport: identities, societies and civilizations,* 1999.

18. Maguire, J. & Stead, D. 'Far Pavilions'?: Cricket Migrants, Foreign Sojourn and Contested Identities. *International Review for the Sociology of Sport.* 31, 1-25. 1996.

19. Maguire, J. & Stead, D. Border Crossings: Soccer Labour Migration and the European Union. *International Review for the Sociology of Sport.* **33,** 59-73. 1998.

20. Olin, K. *Foreign Star Recruit Players as Immigrants: Finnish Basketball as an Illuminative Example.* Research Report: Department of Sociology and Planning for Physical Culture, 1984.

21. Sugden, J. & Tomlinson, A. (eds). *Hosts and champions: Soccer cultures, national identities and the USA World Cup,* 1994.

22. Sugden, J. & Tomlinson, A. *FIFA and the contest for world football,* 1998.

23. Williams, G. 'The road to Wigan Pier revisited: The Migration of Welsh Rugby Talent since 1918'. In: Bale, J. & Maguire, J. (eds). *The Global Sports Arena: Athletic Talent Migration in an Interdependent World,* pp 25-38, 1994.

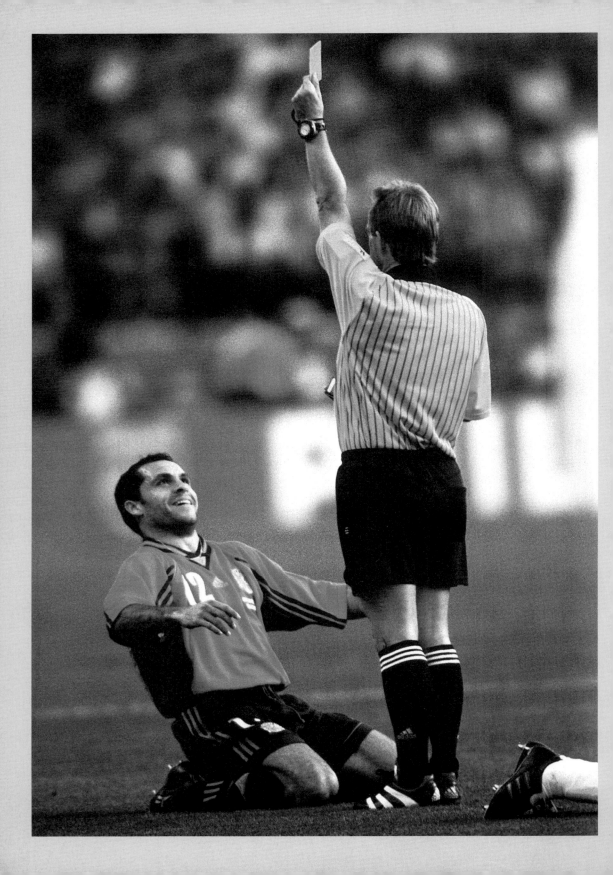

Sport and Morality
The relevance of the traditional Fair Play concept in modern football

Per Nilsson

Synopsis

The purpose of this chapter is to analyse the Fair Play Concept, it's origins and whether the fair play concept is relevant within the modern sport of today. The spreading of rule-breaking is in his paper analysed as a consequence of the historical development of professional sport and as a consequence of a real struggle between different groups of agents linked to different interests within the field of sport.

Introduction

Violence on and around sport arenas as well as drug abuse and cheating have placed the ethics of sport in the public eye. Morality (or more correctly the lack of morality) is a conception often mentioned in these connection.

The concepts of morals and ethics are concerned with principles of right and wrong in relation to human action and character. The word ethics derives from the Greek language (éthiké) and morals from Latin (moralis), but both are concerned with customs and standards of good or right conduct. Very simply expressed, one can say that morals and ethics deal with questions of how people (according to themselves and other people) should act in different situations, and the reasons for their standpoints. In everyday life we usually do not make a separation between morals and ethics. Possibly, morals are more associated with how people should act, while ethics include both the behaviour and the theoretical principles of why some actions are more correct than others (8, 13).

Human standards of what is right and just in behaviour do not exist in a vacuum; such customs and manners must be incorporated in a social context. Morals are formed by social conditions. From this follows that morality can change historically and can differ between sociocultural groups which live under the influence of different social and cultural necessities. Seen in this perspective, ideas of right and wrong conduct, in sport as well as in everyday life, are culturally and socially determined. As a consequence, morality can be regarded as a special form of "social rules" which determine how people perceive, value, experience and act. Morality is what keeps a particular social group or society together, but also separates it from other groups or societies (4). Fair questions to ask, therefore, are what principles of right and good keep sport together and what behaviour patterns create dissension in sport? Is fair play such a guiding norm within sport?

The purpose of this paper is to illustrate the content of the Fair play Concept, it's origin and the historical context in which the term itself was used in the beginning. In the paper I will also try to discuss whether the fair play concept is relevant within modern sport of today and, finally, I will compare the way active football players and referees look at the matter with the official position taken in sports policy.

The Fair Play Concept

As far as we know today the concept of fair play occurred for the first time as a linguistic construction in Shakespeare's classical work "The Life and Death of King John" (1596). In point of language "fair play" then as it does now signified an honourable and loyal way of acting towards written and unwritten rules (12). However, moral codes – with the function of regulating the conditions between two fighting parts and to distinguish more "civilised" groups from others – can be traced much earlier.

For example, the ancient soldier-ethos laid stress upon cunning, courage, loyalty and Victory first. On the other hand the ethos of knights aimed at showing mercy to the opponent and even in certain situations "dissimulate" in order not to debase the adversary (6, 12, 16). In the athletic fair play concept such acting is not acceptable, as everybody are expected to do their best.

It is therefore both right and wrong to say that "fair play" is originating from the ancient Greece or from the medieval games of knights, just to mention a couple of common statements as to the origin of the phenomenon (17). But more important, we are not dealing with an unbroken time-line. The codes of honour mentioned are rather samples of how "attitudes towards morality" are variously expressed at different historical times.

Still, even if "fair play" and "fair" existed as linguistic constructions in the British literature as early as in the end of the 16th century, the concept is usually associated with the sport practised at the English public schools in the 19th century.

What actually happened at these institutions of education was that a number of popular medieval folk games and pastimes, which were originally created by the people as entertainment in connection with feasts, went through a change in meaning and function. Within the public school system these physical exercises, which earlier have been looked upon as vulgar by the privileged layers of society, were taken over by the elite of society and became a pedagogical vehicle for character moulding. As "sports" they were incorporated into the building of character and morals of the British aristocracy.

Moreover, sport became a male culture. At the public schools, the sport of football, for example, was conquered, constructed and confirmed in order to affirm the manly virtues of future leaders (19). Football became an education in stoicism, hardiness, endurance, courage and virility among young men. As a male sport, football was not allowed to be too "weak". If so, the sport would lose its value as a socialisation into manliness. Within the Victorian Great Britain, the well trained body of a man was a symbol of good character and high sexual morality. An ambition to keep the sport tough is therefore apparent in the history of football. But to fulfil its function as a shaper of character, football neither was allowed to be too violent. Within the sport environment, the young man was thought to be tested and refined, but absolutely not be driven to the outskirts of civilisation. Football was thought to be played with dignity in order to secure the social distinction towards the lower strata of society. As a consequence, gains in social prestige were achieved through participation in sports.

In this public school context where sports had become a pedagogical vehicle for character moulding, the amateur rules, including the fair play ideals, served two functions. First, they made a standard for the game. At the time, fair play became a distinctive and powerful moral code of conduct. Fair play was a way of securing a balance between direction to competition and a proper way to behave. Second, these ideals of morality held by the upper social classes functioned as a social distinction towards a more and more threatening working and middle class. Fair play became an attitude towards practice. It was a way to play the game, a way to show clear "role distance" (e.g. not get so carried away by the game so as to forget that it is a game), and to demonstrate disinterest in material gain, as well as to display a will to win, but a will to win within the rules. The amateur rules were in the 19th century used by the privileged layers of society as a way to keep their own sport unaltered and to prohibit other (lower) strata of society to participate in sport (1, 3, 6, 10, 14).

In other words, during the 19th century the fair play concept was given a content of value obviously tied to a certain point of view held by the higher classes of society. The sportsmen (and sportswomen) were not allowed to get too enthusiastic for the games forgetting it all was for fun and for the shaping of character. The game should be carried out under self-control, the same self-control which could be expected by the former leaders of the country (1, 15). An ideal which in many aspects was a product of the liberal ideology of competition. This ideal had itself grown strong in the surrounding society and emphasised obedience to social laws and rules as well as the ethics of hard work, competition, predictability and group-loyalty, i.e. a society without the persuasion towards any important change of it's structure (3, 20). In addition, through the construction of British sport, many of these desirable ideals could be measured, for example through records and competitions (2).

The Fair Play Concept of today

The upholding of many of the traditional fair play ideals has, however, gradually been challenged by a professional view on the game of football, an attitude which has its basis in a transition from amateurism to professionalism. What relevancy then has this traditional fair play concept in the institutional sports of today? According to the ambitions of the Swedish Sport Confederation, the British fair play concept still seems to be extremely valid.

> "'Fair play' in athletics means that the practician shall
> * follow the rules and regulations of athletics
> * show respect for fellow competitors and officials
> * demand the same from oneself as from others, and
> * show a sense of justice and be loyal and generous."
>
> (Source: No 16, 1981 of Minutes from the Swedish Sport Confederation Board)

But how do active sportsmen and the referees look upon fair play? The following results are taken from a study reported 1993 (19). In the study six Swedish Premier League referees were interviewed (open-ended qualitative interviews) and 200 male football players from four different clubs and three different age groups were questioned (both questionnaires and qualitative interviews) about obedience to rules and fair play. The three age groups in the study were elite players from the Premier League in Sweden, youth players at the age of 17-19 and boy players at the age of twelve. To begin with, a number of statements were presented to the players, and the players had to decide how well these statements described the conditions in their own league. Some of the results are shown in Table 1, 2 and 3 respectively.

Table 1. Distribution (%) of answers in the category "Conditions in my own league". Statement: In my team, "victory is the most important".

Level	Quite right	Broadly right	Partially right	Wrong	Do not know
Senior players (n=72)	65	30	3	1	0
Youth players (n=70)	33	40	18	6	3
Boy players (n=56)	9	30	46	11	4

Table 2. Distribution (%) of answers in the category "Conditions in my own league". Statement: In my team it is always important to follow and respect the rules of the game.

Level	Quite right	Broadly right	Partially right	Wrong	Do not know
Senior players (n=72)	56	43	1	0	0
Youth players (n=70)	66	31	3	0	0
Boy players (n=57)	70	28	2	0	0

Table 3. Distribution (%) of answers in the category "Conditions in my own league". Statement: In my team it is OK to pretend being fouled in order to get a free kick.

Level	Quite right	Broadly right	Partially right	Wrong	Do not know
Senior players (n=71)	17	48	22	7	6
Youth players (n=70)	40	31	18	3	7
Boy players (n=56)	4	9	27	52	9

Looking at the answers in Table 1, 2 and 3 it seems as if the players, though to some varying degree, emphasise the importance of winning and the importance of following the rules of football. But how would they answer if they have to choose between the two?

To illuminate that question there was a type of "moral dilemma" constructed where the players had to choose between *breaking the rules and winning or following the rules and losing*. The willingness to follow rules was in that way put into a critical situation. It is hardly worth mentioning that all kinds of behaviour at the sports ground does not demand taking positions of this kind, but in such a situation the choice between the existing norms and valuations are clear in an obvious way. A sample of answers from the groups investigated is illustrated in Table 4. The table summarises how the player himself would act in the situation in question.

Table 4. Distribution (%) of answers in the category "Dilemmas of Morality."

A player gets an obvious opportunity to score. A defender from the other team has a chance to prevent the opponent from scoring, but only by making a foul. (p<0.01)	Senior	Youth	Boys
a) I would commit a foul and play hard even if there is a small risk of hurting the opponent.	29	24	16
b) I would commit a foul and play hard even if there is a great risk of injuring the opponent. Injuries are a part of the game.	7	4	2
c) I would try to stop the opponent by a foul, but in a way that will not risk injuring him.	53	44	44
d) I would try to stop the opponent at any price, for example by knocking or kicking him down, even though he may be injured.	0	1	2
e) I would play fair even if it does not prevent the opponent from scoring.	11	16	35
f) Other alternative (respondents own).	0	10	2
Total	100	100	100

The answers to this "moral dilemma" show a far more forgiving attitude to disobedience of rules than was apparent in Table 1, 2 and 3. It is therefore a considerable difference between discussing the importance of following rules in general versus in specific situations where the players have to weigh various actions against each other. The answers also verify that the players (in varying degrees) have developed an attitude towards rules and fair play indicating that in specific situations it is considered excusable and fair to break the rules of football. It should be mentioned, though, that the groups investigated disassociated themselves from the most excessive assaults and from injuring an opponent intentionally.

How then does, the referees value the importance of following the rules of the game? The referees' responsibility is, on behalf of the officials (e.g. The Swedish Football Confederation), to execute and preserve the formal rules in practice. This task is, however, complicated by the fact that the referees beside their role as "guardians of the law" also at the same time are part of the football practice, and as a consequence of this also will be influenced by the conditions of the game.

Which consequences follow from this "middle position"? How should a "good referee" behave, according to the referees' own opinion? This is a quotation from the interviews:

> *Q: What do you think is the most important obligation of the referee?*
> *A: The longer I have been active as a football referee, the clearer it is to me that my job is to create a good atmosphere on the field, and the behaviour of the referee (e.g. the body language) is as important as the decisions. Then you should realise that football is played for the sake of the teams. The referee should never be allowed to play a leading part. As a referee you are some kind of an assistant. For example, you have to put the rules into practice. If you stick too closely to the formal rules there will be far too many interruptions. Nobody wants it that way. You have to find a way to lead the match without too many breaks. You have to find a way that is acceptable. You can't let everything go, neither can you take measure of all the faults.*
> *Q: You must search for a balance?*
> *A: Yes, there has to be flexibility in the interpretation of the rules.*

This ambiguity, that is obvious in this referee's attitude towards rule observance, should not be interpreted – or understood – as a result of individual and personal shortcomings, but primarily as a consequence of those different demands which are placed upon the referees from various other groups within the social field of football (18). The media and the spectators, for example, want to have an exciting and entertaining play without too many breaks, the players and their clubs want glory, success and fame, and The Swedish Football Association, finally, wants the play on the field to be in accordance with the traditional fair play idea (at least as long as there still are preconditions to develop an internationally competitive football within the country).

The development of modern sport

How should one explain this dispositions towards practice expressed by the players and the position taken by the referees? Why is there such a big gap between ideals and reality? An important starting point is that the way the players and referees think and act always has to be related to the practice of which they are a part. With a reference to established historical and sociological literature about sport, it could be stated that the western competitive sports, in an reflexive process with the surrounding society during the 19th and 20th centuries, have developed towards a more obvious degree of seriousness and direction towards results (3, 5, 7). The development points towards a professional sport, more and more removing from the old amateur ideals. Sport on professional level tends to be an activity more and more aiming at satisfying the needs of the sponsors, media and spectators rather than the participants. The increasing financial and social meaning of victory leads to a more instrumental behaviour within (and without) the limits of the rules (9).

The description of the development of sports mentioned above – the increasing international competition, the increasing national significance of elite sports and the market economical situations which raise the winner's value compared to the other competitors – explains why the attitudes towards fair play and rule breaking within sport have changed over time. But in order to understand the variations of how the players, the referees and the National Sport Confederation look upon rules and fair play, it is necessary to mention something about the nature of the rules.

To summarise, the task of the rules is on the one hand to state and emphasise the specific marks that characterise a certain sport (i.e. to define within which activity one should compete) and on the other hand to realise a direction of will about what is needed to be preserved, reinforced or forbidden in order to guarantee that the "right sport" survives. This means of course that various groups of agents with different interests in the game develop different attitudes towards the application of rules and to what is to be considered fair play. It is important, however, to see this not only as a philosophical discussion about "the essence of the sport" or as a private question of morality. At a high degree, these different attitudes also represent a real struggle between different groups of agents with different possibilities to mobilise resources for the shaping of competitive sports in the future. The result is a dialectic process where unwanted tendencies among players (for example violence an drug abuse) lead to sharpened rules, increased control, information campaigns, etc. from the confederations - actions and changes which the participants have to follow, or at least relate themselves to (5, 11). The valid rules may therefore be considered a mean as well as a result of a struggle between various groups of agents within a social field of competition (1).

This means that the pattern of thinking and acting incorporated within the practice of the sports by individuals and groups are dependent on the position of the individual or group within a social field of competition, as well as the historical development of sports and the organisational construction.

Conclusion

The purpose in this paper was to analyse the Fair Play Concept, it's origins and the various historical contexts in which the term have been used. The analysis shows that different moral codes with different content can be traced to particular historical and geographical contexts. Having said that, "fair play" and "fair" as linguistic constructions are usually associated with the sport practised at the British public schools in the 19th century. In addition, in this paper I have discussed whether the fair play concept is relevant within the modern sport of today. In that context, the spreading of rule-breaking has been seen as a consequence of the historical development of professional sport and as a consequence of a real struggle between different groups of agents linked to different interests within the field of sport.

References

1. Bourdieu, P. Sport and Social Class. *Social Science Information* (SAGE Publications), Vol. 17, No. 6, p.p. 819-840, 1978.
2. Crosset, T. Masculinity, Sexuality, and the Development of Early Modern Sport. In Messner, M. & Sabo, D.F. (eds.) *Sport, Men and the Gender Order. Critical Feminist Perspectives.* Human Kinetics Books, Champaign, Illinois, pp 45-54, 1990.
3. Dunning, E. & Sheard, K. *Barbarians, Gentlemen and Players. A Sociological Study of the Development of Rugby Football.* Oxford, Martin Robertson, 1979.
4. Durkheim, E. *Durkheim. Essays on morals and education.* Routledge & Kegan Paul, London, 1979.
5. Gruneau, R. *Class, Sports, and Social Development.* The University of Massachusetts Press, Amherst, 1983.
6. Guttman, A. Ursprunge, Soziale Basis und Zukunft des Fair Play. *Sportwissenschaft,* 1978, Vol. 1, p.p. 1-19, 1978.
7. Guttman, A. *From Ritual to Record. The Nature of Modern Sports.* Columbia University Press, New York, 1979.
8. Hedin, C. *Etikens grunder. En vägledning bland värden och normer.* HLS Förlag, 1993.
9. Heinilä, K. The Totalization Process in International Sport. *Sportwissenschaft,* Vol. 3, p.p. 235-254, 1982.
10. Holt, R. *Sport and the British. A Modern History.* Oxford Studies in Social History. Clarendon Press, 1989.
11. Kew, F. Contested Rules: an explanation of how games change. *International Review for the Sociology of Sport,* Vol. 22, p.p. 122-135, 1987.
12. Lipponski, W. *Recognizing the Celts: Some remarks on the British Origins of the Modern Fair Play Concept.* Paper presented at the 8th International Scientific Congress for Students, Budapest, 1988.
13. Loland, S. *Fair play i idrettskonkurranser – et moraliskt normsystem.* Doktoravhandling, Norges Idrettshögskole, 1989.
14. Mangan, J.A. *Athleticism in the Victorian and Edwardian public school. The Emergence and Consolidation of an Educational Ideology.* The Falmer Press, London, 1981.
15. Mangan, J.A. *The Games Ethic and Imperialism. Aspects of the Diffusion of an Ideal.* Viking, Middlesex, 1986.
16. Mc Intosh, P. *Fair Play. Ethics in Sport and Education.* Heineman, London, 1979.
17. Nilsson, P. Fair play inom den moderna tävlingsidrotten – exemplet fotboll. *SVEBI:s Årsbok 1990. Aktuell svensk beteendevetenskaplig idrottsforskning, Lund,* 1990.
18. Nilsson, P. Bra fotboll – Vad är det? *SVEBI:s Årsbok 1991. Aktuell svensk beteendevetenskaplig idrottsforskning, Lund,* 1991.
19. Nilsson, P. *Fotbollen och moralen. En studie av fyra allsvenska fotbollsföreningar.* HLS Förlag, Stockholm, 1993.
20. Rigauer, B. *Sport and Work.* Columbia University Press, New York, 1981.

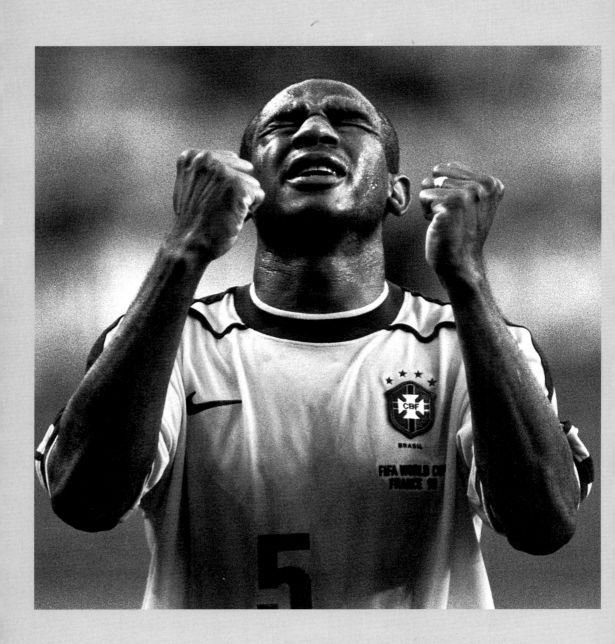

Soccer and Emotion: Enhancing or Impairing Performance?

Yuri L. Hanin

Synopsis

The Individual Zones of Optimal Functioning (IZOF) model is proposed as a framework to describe and explain emotion-performance relationships in skilled soccer players. The main features of the IZOF model include: a multidimensional conception of performance related states, a categorization of emotion content, stepwise procedures for individualized emotion profiling, and prediction of individual and team performance based on the in-out of the zone notion. Applications aim to improve players' awareness of the role of subjective emotional experiences through a detailed feedback emphasizing individuality that enhances team's strengths.

Introduction

Soccer is an important area of research and consultancy that involves sociological, psychological, physiological, biomechanical and pedagogical aspects that are usually addressed separately. However, factors that enhance or impair individual or team performance present a key perspective that could be taken as a basis for integrating available knowledge about the game of football, about the players, coaches, management, and specific environment. Thus, we could benefit from looking at possible connections and an inter- and multidisciplinary overlap that might provide some promising developments for joint efforts in future research and applications.

Therefore, the goal of the present paper is to examine subjective emotional experiences in skilled soccer players that can have either beneficial or detrimental effects on individual (or team) performance. Conceptually, this approach is based on the Individual Zones of Optimal Functioning (IZOF) model developed as an idiographic (individual-oriented) alternative to the study of emotions in elite sport (13). Empirically, the paper is based on extensive practical experiences in individualized assessment, monitoring and interventions during a 3-year on-going project with the Finnish Olympic soccer team.

After a brief overview of the IZOF model and assessment procedures using individualized mood scales, selected empirical findings on patterns of optimal and dysfunctional emotions and emotion-performance relationships in skilled soccer players will be described. Implications and future directions for interdisciplinary research and consultancy for extending the IZOF model will be suggested.

The IZOF Model

The IZOF model, developed in top sports setting, combines within – and between – individual analyses of subjective emotional experiences related to individually optimal and poor performances. The main emphasis in the model is on enhancing consistency of an athlete's successful performance. Initially, the IZOF model was used to study optimal pre-competition anxiety and patterns of positive and negative emotions or affect (PNA) in different sports (6, 7, 8, 13). As applied to pre-competition anxiety, this approach indicates that each athlete has an individually optimal intensity level that can be high, moderate, or low and zones of optimal anxiety enhancing an athlete's performance. Successful performance occurs when current precompetition anxiety is near or within the individually optimal intensity zones. When pre-competition anxiety falls outside the zones, i.e., higher or lower, individual performance usually deteriorates. In team sports setting, such as soccer, ice-hockey, rowing, etc. the findings about the individual nature of optimal and dysfunctional emotions are especially relevant due to the intensive interpersonal and intragroup influences.

Recently several new features were developed in the IZOF model extended to the study of positive and negative emotions enhancing and impairing individual performance. First, the framework of five basic dimensions (form, content, intensity, time and context) for the systems description of emotions as a part of an individual's performance-related psychobiosocial working state was proposed. Second, emotion content was conceptualized within the framework of two combined factors: *hedonic tone* (pleasant-unpleasant) and *functional impact* (optimal-dysfunctional). Thus, four global content categories were derived: positive, pleasant, and functionally optimal emotions (P+); negative, unpleasant, and functionally optimal emotions (N+); positive, pleasant, and dysfunctional emotions (P-); and negative, unpleasant, and dysfunctional emotions (N-). Third, the prediction of individually successful, average or poor performance is based on the "in-out of the zone" principle. Thus, a player's current (or anticipatory) emotional state is first described in terms of individually relevant emotion content and then emotion intensity is contrasted with the previously established individually optimal and dysfunctional intensity zones. High probability of successful performance is expected when emotion intensity is within the optimal zones and outside nonoptimal ranges. Fourth, step-wise assessment procedures were developed to generate: (a) optimal and nonoptimal emotion profiles and (b) recall, current, and anticipatory measures on individualized context-specific self-rating scales with athlete-generated items. These provided tools for the accurate prediction of individual emotion-performance relationships and post-performance analysis. Based on such assessments, the individualized intervention procedures matching individual's needs and task specifics are then developed.

Emotion Patterns in Skilled Soccer Players

Most of the IZOF research at this point is focused on the prototype analysis of the content and intensity of positive and negative emotions that are helpful and harmful for individual and team performance. This approach challenges a widespread myth implied in sport psychology interventions based on inverted-U hypothesis or on the multidimensional anxiety theory. Specifically, it shows that positive emotions, e.g., *calm, confident, relaxed, joyful,* are not always functionally optimal, whereas negative emotions, e.g., *angry, dissatisfied, nervous,* are not always dysfunctional for performance. Appraisals of current situation are the key cognitive processes that determine the generation of both pleasant and unpleasant emotions. However, their impact on performance will be different if challenge (or threat) appraisal pattern is reversed into gain (or loss) pattern prematurely during performance when the task is not completed. Moreover, strong emotions are usually motivational and help to stay focused on the task and to maintain an adequate effort level, whereas weak emotions are de-motivational and usually result in diminished (or even discontinued) effort and less than effective focus (13, 14). Specific situational context of the game in soccer and team dynamics is also important as the basis of the interpretation of whether an emotion is functional or dysfunctional. Therefore, it is crucial to first identify emotions really experienced by athletes and then to examine their functional impact in different players prior to and during successful and poor performance. However, a detailed functional analysis requires an accurate description of emotion content and emotion intensity changing over time across different contexts.

Emotion Content in Soccer Players

There are several options in describing emotion content in skilled soccer players. For instance, based on existing conceptualizations of emotion, we could describe emotional experiences of players in terms of global affect (positive and negative emotions) or as single, discrete or primary emotions (anxiety, anger, fun, self-confidence). There are dozens of normative, standardized emotion or mood scales that can be used to describe how players feel before, during or after the game (or practices). Most popular scales developed in non-sport settings are Spielberger et al's (21) State-Trait-Anxiety Inventory (STAI), Profile of Mood State (POMS), and Watson and Tellegen's (26) Positive and Negative Affect Schedule (PANAS). Sport-specific scales include Martens et al's (18) Competitive State Anxiety Inventory (CSAI-2) and Smith et al's (20) Sports Anxiety Scale (SAS).

One problem with these psychometric normative (group–oriented) scales is that they have a "fixed" content (a pool of researcher-generated items) that usually implies the same psychological meaning of emotion descriptors for all athletes. Moreover, in most cases, it is not known to what extent emotion content assessed with the normative scales reflects players' idiosyncratic subjective experiences related to successful and poor performances.

Two recent studies involving 50 skilled soccer players and 46 ice-hockey players provide empirical evidence comparing the content of emotion items in normative, standardized scales and individual emotional experiences as reflected in athlete-generated descriptors (23, 24). Specifically, it was found that about 80-85% of emotion content (items) relevant for the individual players is not included in the standardized scales. In other words, a researcher or a practitioner using these scales should be aware of the fact that more than 80% of emotional content of real performance-related subjective experiences will simply not be measured at all.

Another option in the description of emotion patterns in soccer is to use the individualized scales with athlete-generated items that are based directly on players' awareness of their past performance experiences. The IZOF framework proposes two combined principles for the individualized assessments. First, athletes are selecting (generating) items within the framework of four global categories: positive-optimal (P+), negative-optimal (N+), negative-dysfunctional (N-), and positive-dysfunctional (P-). Thus an athlete is "forced" to report his or her past subjective experiences (both pleasant and unpleasant) in terms of how helpful or harmful they were for individual performance. However, it is important that the idiosyncratic items are selected within these four categories without any restriction or limitation. As a first step to the prototype description of emotion in soccer (or any other sport), it seems to be the best strategy, because individually generated items can then be content analyzed and classified into other content categories (anxiety, anger, frustration, distress, etc.). Additionally, the idea was to emphasize a holistic nature of self-ratings and to generate performance-related content for more detailed analysis.

Generating Individualized Emotion Descriptors

The content of individually optimal and nonoptimal emotion patterns in games (and practices) is assessed using the idiographic recall method suggested by Hanin (10, 11). This method identifies subjectively meaningful positive and negative emotions in terms of the individual's past performance history and significant emotional experiences. In idiographic recall, athletes generate individually relevant emotion words that best describe their optimal (helpful) and dysfunctional (harmful) positive and negative emotions. To help athletes to generate individual items, the emotion stimulus list is used and it included positive and negative emotions typically experienced in performance. The English version of the emotion stimulus list was compiled through selection and revision of items from the 10 global PNA scales described by Watson and Tellegen (27). These items were then translated into Finnish, and three judges evaluated the item content by selecting the most appropriate synonyms used in current spoken Finnish. The final version of the emotion list included 40 positive emotions and 37 negative emotions. Examples of positive affect items include *active, calm, confident, pleased, determined, excited.* Negative affect items include *nervous, angry, annoyed, irritated, dissatisfied,* and *uncertain.*

Recall scaling includes several steps. First, optimal emotion patterns are identified. Athletes, using the emotion stimulus list, select 4 or 5 positive and then 4 or 5 negative items that best describe their emotions related to individually successful performances in the past. Then dysfunctional emotion patterns are identified by selecting 4 or 5 positive and 4 or 5 negative items that describe their emotions related to individually unsuccessful performances. In order to elicit a pattern, repeated experiences on several occasions are emphasized rather than one specific situation. Athletes use the emotion stimulus list to generate individually relevant positive and negative descriptors and can also add emotion words of their own choice. Step-wise procedures and the IZOF

Table 1

Top ten positive optimal (P+) and dysfunctional (P-) emotions in soccer

Optimal positive emotions	Dysfunctional positive emotions
Latautunut .... charged	Huoleton .... easy-going
Energinen .... energetic	Mukava .... comfortable
Motivoitunut .... motivated	Tyyni .... tranquil
Luottavainen .... confident	Peloton .... fearless
Sähäkkä .... alert	Iki-ihastunut .... overjoyed
Jännitynyt .... excited	Kiva .... nice
Varma .... certain	Vilkas .... animated
Rihkea .... brave	Varma .... certain
Määrätietoinen .... purposeful	Tyytyväinen .... satisfied
Innostunut .... enthusiastic	Hurmioitunut .... exalted

Table 2

Top ten negative optimal (N+) and dysfunctional (N-) emotions in soccer

Optimal negative emotions	Dysfunctional negative emotions
Jännitynyt .... excited	Väsynyt .... tired
Tyytymätön .... dissatisfied	Haluton .... unwilling
Hyökkäävä .... attacking	Epävarma .... uncertain
Kiihkeä .... vehement	Vellto .... sluggish
Kiivas .... intense	Laiska .... lazy
Hermostunut .... nervous	Murhellinen .... sorrowful
Ärtynyt .... irritated	Onneton .... unhappy
Ärsyyntynyt .... provoked	Masentunut .... depressed
Rauhaton .... restless	Pelokas .... afraid
Levoton .... uneasy	Uupunut .... exhausted

forms are described in Hanin (10, 14). (Paper and pencil and computerized versions of the procedure are available in English, Finnish, Spanish, Norwegian, Polish, Portuguese, and Russian).

Let us say, a soccer player A, based on past experiences, selected five positive-optimal emotions *(motivated, charged, brisk, resolute, active)*, two negative-optimal *(vehement, attacking)*, three positive-dysfunctional *(calm, comfortable, pleasant)*, and four negative-dysfunctional *(tired, sad, dispirited, distressed)*. This is an individualized set of emotion content that is relevant for this particular athlete and is related to the game context in general. In contrast, a player B, might select quite different emotions: four positive-optimal emotions *(motivated, purposeful, willing, excited)*, three negative-optimal *(irritated, dissatisfied, tense)*, four positive-dysfunctional *(good, glad, satisfied, fearless)*, and five negative-dysfunctional *(unhappy, dejected, lazy, tired, sluggish)*. Each player's emotion descriptors reflect their unique experiences in coping with successful or poor performance situations. Therefore, some of the selected emotions within the four global categories are different, whereas others are similar. However, as a first step in the analysis of emotion content it is more important to identify specific, idiosyncratic, and functionally relevant emotions than to simply describe interindividual difference on set of descriptors that may not be relevant to either of these two players. On the other hand, if we look at the list of all emotion items selected (or not selected) by several or all players in the team, we can get a big picture of emotion prototypes: "core" or most selected emotions, moderately selected and idiosyncratic emotions (Hanin & Syrjä, 1995a & 1999b). For instance, top ten positive and negative emotions within each of the four global categories that were selected most often by skilled soccer players are reported in Tables 1 and 2

These emotion descriptors characterize "typical" (aggregated) emotions experienced by skilled players in different game situations based on direct personal experiences and their awareness of these experiences. However, it is also important to realize that these group data cannot be applied directly to monitor emotional dynamics in a particular player or a particular team. That would require a person-oriented (or team-oriented) individualized emotion profiling aimed to identify an individual's (or team's) change, growth, and development. Furthermore, based only on these individual data, it is possible to examine to what extent partners or players performing different functions are similar or different in their emotional response and in the way they use their resources. Additionally, if a coach is working with a new team it

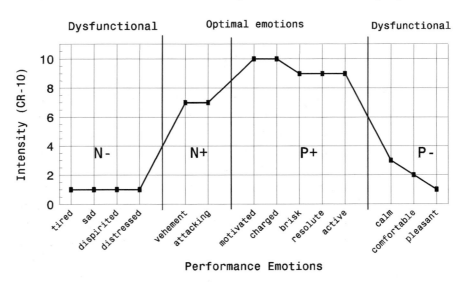

Fig. 1 Individualized pre-game emotion profile of a soccer player A Explanations in the text.

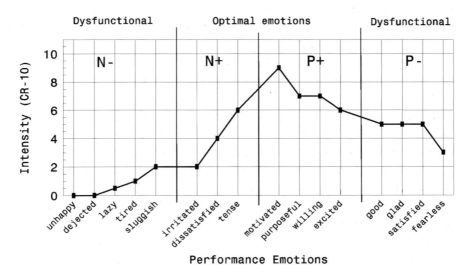

Fig. 2 Individualized pre-game emotion profile of a soccer player B Explanations in the text.

might be useful to be aware of the emotion patterns in new players invited to the team.

Emotion Intensity in Soccer Players

Although the content of emotions experienced before and during games is crucial for the functional interpretation of emotional impact on performance, content alone is not sufficient. Another dimension is the optimal and dysfunctional intensity (ranges or zones) of specific emotions within each of the four global categories. Therefore, in our research and consultancy work, we used the Borg's (1, 2) Category Ratio (CR-10) scale that rates intensity within the range from 0 (nothing at all) to 10 and # (maximal possible) (13, 15, 16, 17, 25). In our previous example with players A and B, each emotion item was rated for intensity before a successful game. As shown in Fig. 1 and 2, even though the sets of items selected by players A and B are different, their individualized emotion profiles form what is termed "IZOF-iceberg" profiles. It is noteworthy that a relatively high intensity in optimal emotions located in the middle (P+ and N+) in the IZOF-iceberg profile is accompanied by a low intensity in dysfunctional items located by the sides (N- and P-). Therefore, the IZOF-emotion iceberg profile is a deliberately constructed visual representation of an interactive (additive) effect of high intensity optimal, enhancing and low intensity dysfunctional, impairing emotions upon individual performance.

On the other hand, if the limitation of aggregated scores/profiles is clearly recognized they can be used for more general and descriptive purposes (e.g. to identify trends in emotion intensity patterns, to develop "soccer" IZOF-emotion iceberg profile, to compare players of different skill level, age, and gender). It is important to realize that, the content of athlete-generated emotion descriptors in aggregated scales is more sports-specific than the content of researcher-generated items in existing normative scales. Two examples illustrating the possibility of using aggregated scores in combination with individualized scales are reported below.

First, emotion intensity patterns can be described also at the group level across the four global categories by aggregating individual items. For instance, the intensity of optimal (P+ = 6.5, N+ = 4.1) and dys-

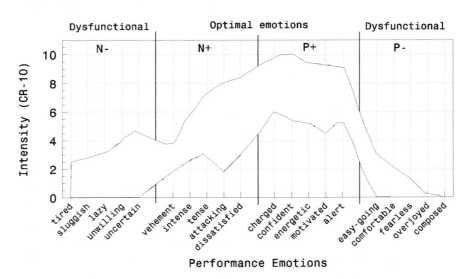

Fig. 3 IZOF-emotion iceberg in soccer based on top five emotions selected by the players (N=29)

functional (P- = 4.3, N- = 6.0) emotions in pre-match situations in 25 Olympic level soccer players reflects the same interactive relation-ships that are found at the individual level (Hanin & Syrjä, 1995a). These findings were replicated in a sample of 25 young skilled soccer players and the pre-match intensity of optimal (P+ = 6.5, N+ = 4.5) and dysfunctional (P- = 7.4, N- = 7.5) emotions were nearly the same (19).

Second, it is possible for illustrative and descriptive purposes to develop an aggregated "soccer" IZOF-emotion iceberg profile. The data from 29 highly skilled soccer players were used to identify top five (mostly selected by soccer players) emotions in each of the four emotion categories. Aggregated optimal intensity zones for enhancing (P+N+) items located in the middle and impairing (P-N-) items located by the sides form a bell-shaped or iceberg emotion profile (Fig. 3). Being in the optimal zones visually reflects an interaction of high enhan-cing and low impairing effects of emotions and thus a high probability of successful performance. Deviations from the optimal zones indicate to some areas that might need either problem – or emotion – coping.

It is interesting that the visual representation of interaction effect by the IZOF-iceberg profile is the same for both individual and the group level data. In all cases, successful performance is accompanied by an IZOF-iceberg, whereas poor performance is associated with the "flat" iceberg or shallow profile.

Individualized Emotion Scales and IZOF-iceberg

A set of individually selected emotion items is used in repeated assess-ments of current, or past (recalled), or anticipated emotional states. However, these individualized emotion scales with items reflecting optimal and dysfunctional impact on performance, are useful not only for description but also for prediction of performance and for post-performance analysis. Content validity of these scales is established through the process of their construction and generation of individually relevant items. However, reliability of the scales can be established by examining how consistent athlete's ratings are in repeated assessments.

A series of studies was undertaken to examine reliability (intraindi-vidual alphas) and the accuracy of anticipatory, current, and recall measures of emotion using individualized emotion scales (17). The reliability of the individualized emotion scales was established intraindividually by calculating Cronbach alpha-coefficients for each subscale. The highest internal consistency was observed in positive and negative facilitating (P+N+) items: alpha M = .90, SD = .04, ranging from 0.82 to 0.96. In positive-optimal (P+) items alpha M = .86, SD = .08, ranging from .66 to .99, whereas in negative-optimal (N+) items alpha M = .83, SD = 0.13, ranging from .57 to .96. In subscales with positive-dysfunctional (P-) and negative-dysfunctional (N-) items alphas M = .79 (SD = .16, with a range of .44 to .99), and .54 (SD = .21, with a range of .26 to .96), respectively. In dysfunctional positive and negative (P-N-) items, alpha M = .76, SD = .13, ranging from .44 to .96. Lower internal consistency was obtained for the total PNA scale: alpha M = .57, SD = .14, ranging from .35 to.73.

It should be noted that high consistency of skilled players' ratings in repeated intraindividual assessments indicates that the individualized emotion scales and the IZOF-based procedures are reliable. Moreover, intraindividual alphas can also serve as indirect indicators of a player's awareness of own subjective experiences and ability to report them. Athletes of lower skill level or lacking in sport experience could be less consistent in their self-assessments. However, with repeated assessments and increased awareness, the consistency and accuracy of the ratings increase. Thus, alphas could be used not only to assess intraindividual reliability of the individualized emotion scale, but also to evaluate indirectly a player's awareness of the subjective emotional experiences related to successful and poor performances. Additionally, content (face) validity or relevancy of individually selected items is re-examined and more accurate emotion descriptors can be generated based on an athlete's enhanced awareness.

Based on the accuracy of recalls and prediction scores compared with actual assessments, the procedures matching team's routines and preparation patterns were developed to avoid unnecessary or distracting assessments on the day prior to the international games. Additionally, by changing instructions it was possible to use individualized emotion scales in the assessment of the impact of the climate and atmosphere in the club and the national teams upon player's performance, as well as coach's and interplayer influences.

Emotion-Performance Relationships in Soccer Players

The second direction of the IZOF-based research aims to test the in-out of the zone principle by examining the within-individual dynamics of emotions before, during, and after performance in skilled and in junior soccer players (13, 25). Here, the impact of individually optimal and dysfunctional emotions upon athletic performance is examined by contrasting current (or anticipatory) intensities of each emotion in the emotion profile with the previously established optimal and dysfunctional zones.

IZOF-based Predictions of Performance

As mentioned earlier, the IZOF emotion-iceberg profile visually represent an interactive (additive) effect of optimal (positive and negative) and dysfunctional (positive and negative) emotions. The main emphasis here is on the functional meaning of individually selected and performance-related emotions, rather than on their hedonic tone (positivity versus negativity) as an indicator of general well being. In contrast, the well known POMS-iceberg compares a fixed positive dimension *(vigour)* and a fixed negative dimension *(anger, tension, confusion, fatigue, depression)* which are functionally implied to be similar for all athletes. The prominence of optimal (both positive and negative emotions) over dysfunctional (positive and negative) emotions in the IZOF emotion iceberg reflects the fundamental fact that during the sporting activity typically mixed emotions are experienced and can produce a mixed effect. Optimal emotions are enhancing performance by providing energy for effort and skills for its allocation (the right focus). Dysfunctional emotions impair performance by distracting resources to task-irrelevant cues, and by de-mobilization efforts. In other words, emotions enhancing and impairing individual performance are functionally related with motivational, volitional, and cognitive processes. Although, specific relationships between these processes are to be established by future researchers, the total interactive impact of emotions on performance can be derived from two separate (enhancing [+] and impairing [-]) emotion effects:

(1) Best performance = (High [+]) + (Low [-])
(2) Average performance = (High [+]) + (High [-])
(3) Average performance = (Low [+]) + (Low [-])
(4) Poor performance = (Low [+]) + (High [-])

Selected Empirical Findings

The validity of the in-out of the zone notion and practical utility of the above predictions were tested empirically in several studies involving junior and Olympic level soccer players (11, 12, 15, 19, 25) and rugby and ice-hockey players (3, 16). A brief overview of the selected soccer studies will be given below in the sections that follow.

The studies confirmed the assumptions about the interactive (additive) effects of enhancing and impairing emotions upon athletic performance, especially in games, as contrasted with practices. Specifically, in games the differences in emotion intensity deviations before and during performance were significant and in the predicted direction. Successful players, as compared to average and poor performance players, were closer to optimal and outside of dysfunctional zones. After the games all differences, except for negative-optimal and positive-dysfunctional emotions, were significant (Kruskal-Wallis test). In practices significant differences in the predicted direction (except, for positive-dysfunctional and total deviations from the zones) were observed only during but not before the performance.

Similar findings were obtained by computing correlations between total deviations of emotion items from the zones and individual performance. In games predicted relationships were observed in 81,0 % of all 21 cases, with more significant correlations for deviation from dysfunctional zones, optimal zones, negative-dysfunctional emotions and the total interactive deviation. During performance, significant correlations were found for deviation from positive-optimal emotion zones ($r = -0.57$, $p<0.01$), negative-dysfunctional zones ($r = 0.28$, $p<0.01$), total optimal zones ($r = -0.38$, $p<0.01$), and combined effects ($r = 0.47$, $p<0.01$). The results of regression analysis indicated that joint impact of ineffective (negative) and effective (positive) emotions accounted for 41.8 % ($F=23.0$, $p<0.01$) of variance and deviations from negative-dysfunctional alone accounted for 34.0% of variance ($F=33.5$, $p<0.01$) in the games. In practices 31.6% of variance in performance was explained by joint impact of positive-optimal and negative-dysfunctional emotions (F = 20.3, p<0.01), whereas deviations from the positive-optimal emotion zones alone explained 26.7 % of variance (F = 32.5, p<0.01).

The results of the Friedman test indicated that emotion intensity (P+, N+, P-, N-, P+N+, P-N-, and P+N+P-N-) before, during and after performance change over time, however, differently in successful and poor performance groups. For instance, poor performance players were outside their optimal zones already before the game. And, even if they managed to enter their optimal emotion zones spontaneously during performance, they still failed to maintain it. After the game their emotion ratings dropped dramatically. Thus in poor performance group emotion change over time was observed in 88.2 % of all cases. On the other hand, successful players were closer to their optimal emotion patterns and outside dysfunctional patterns already before the game. Moreover, they managed to maintain their optimal emotions until the task was completed. As a result, the emotion change over time in successful performance group was also observed but less often than in poor performance group (37.5 %). However, in successful performance group players sometimes stayed in the optimal emotional state even after the game which might create a problem for their adequate recovery. Finally, it was found that emotions not only influenced players' performance but also were influenced by their subsequent performance. In other words, the direction of emotion-performance relationship was reciprocal and changed over time.

In conclusion, these findings indicate that players who experienced optimal emotions of sufficient intensity and were low on intensity in dysfunctional emotions (high [+] and low [-] effects), usually performed up to their potential. In contrast, players with emotion intensities in the high [+] and high [-], low [+] and low [-], or low [+] and high [-] effect zones were less than successful. In other words, the in-out of the zone notion proved to be a valid principle that accounted for the interaction effect of emotions with functionally different impact.

These findings were also used qualitatively to predict each player's psychological readiness for a very important international match of the Finnish (U-21) Olympic team. Two days before the game, players' current emotional states were assessed and contrasted with their individually optimal emotion profiles. Most players for several reasons (successful games in the National championships, good camp and accommodation) were feeling too self-confident and comfortable, thus not ready to perform up to their potential. Head coach discussed the situation with the players explaining the findings obtained earlier with this team and other teams. This has changed players' attitudes to the forthcoming match and the entire atmosphere in the team. As a result, players became more focused, motivated and prepared much better for the game and a draw (1:1) with a much stronger opponent was equal to victory.

Finally, it is important to realize that both the quantitative and qualitative findings reported above describe mainly the impact of optimal and dysfunctional emotions on individual performance in team setting. The IZOF model, however, provides tools for the extension of this initial emphasis to the optimal performance of the entire team through the analysis of the role of group and interpersonal factors. For instance, it is important to establish emotion profiles of the key players and the dynamics of their emotion-motivational states when the team is winning or losing. Then it is possibly to identify optimal communication patterns that lead to optimal emotional states in the team (9), especially, during tournaments and across the entire season.

Implications and Applications

Both directions of research briefly described, at least cross-sectionally and at the level of sporting activity, provide a relatively complete description of emotional impact on individual and team performance in soccer players. What is missing is the analysis of the situational dynamics of emotion during performance and the reciprocity of emotion-performance relationships. This aspect of emotion-performance relationships is being investigated in a series of studies that are under way (14, 22).

From an applied perspective, the IZOF-based assessment package provides a unique opportunity for giving detailed feedback both to players and coaches. This information is then fitted into the preparation of the team and goal-setting for individual players (or partners) in the particular match. However, it is also important to emphasize that IZOF assessments are not merely focused on the development of the individualized emotion scales and emotion profiling. These procedures also provide a tool to indirectly structure, re-structure, and enhance an individual's awareness and acceptance of the subjective emotional experiences. Self-assessments usually trigger players thinking about their practices, preparation routines, their performance and experiences in terms of consistently optimal and dysfunctional effects. This process leads to self-programming the right attitudes to the game and better understanding of the key factors that help to enter the optimal zones and keep this individually effective focus during the game. Moreover, as soon as dysfunctional emotions are recognized, this awareness on the part of players and a coach leads to new strategies of predicting and coping with different distractions. At the same time, communication between the players and the coach as well as the team's emotional climate can improve dramatically (4, 5, 7, 9). Optimal communication in the soccer team is especially important for effective regulation of optimal emotional states in key players affecting the rest of the team. All these lead to a marked shift of focus to the mastery orientation, high quality practices, players' own impact and responsibility resulting in a more mature attitude to all they are doing to grow both personally and professionally.

Future Directions

Based on applied and action-oriented research and consultancy with skilled soccer players, several directions in the application of the IZOF model in soccer can be suggested. These include an in-depth analysis of players' individual strengths and limitations (performance profiling), patterns of active recovery from demanding games during the season, team building through better awareness of own optimal patterns and those of teammates. A new challenge for researchers and practitioners would be to examine the key emotion factors for consistent excellency in performance of individual players and that of the team. For instance, it is crucial for a coach to know how the key players in the team can affect each other optimal and dysfunctional zones prior to, during and after the game. The most important factor here might be coach's and players' interpersonal influences and status-role relationships.

Certain implications that bear directly on future inter- and multidisciplinary emphasis should be also mentioned. First, this paper emphasized only emotional (affective) functioning and the ways to assess and monitor optimal and dysfunctional emotions. Future research should include other modalities of the psychobiosocial state, such as motivational, cognitive, somatic, psychomotor, performance and communicative components.

For instance, cognitive and motivational functioning are the next components that can significantly enrich working states profiles. Interestingly enough, several items in the emotion profiles generated by players included descriptors with cognitive *(alert, attentive, concentrated)* and motivational *(willing, motivated, interested, enthusiastic)* content. In other words, players themselves are more holistic in describing how they feel prior to or during the game. Therefore, further research is clearly indicated in order to develop, for instance, individualized emotional-motivational or emotional-somatic-motor behavioral profiles following the procedures already described. This line of research might result in the development of the IZOF based psychobiosocial profiles in soccer players.

From the interdisciplinary perspective of great interest in future studies is the somatic dimension. However, the description of somatic dimension (somatic profiling) is not enough. More important physiologically would be a functional interpretation of the emotion profiles in terms of two basic functions (energy mobilization and energy utilization). Physiological monitoring of responses during the game can be related to subjective emotional experiences using stimulated recall with individualized emotion scales through the analysis of videos of game performance.

Another challenge for both researchers (e.g. sport psychologists and biomechanics) and practitioners would be the individualized description of the performance process. Preliminary findings indicate that IZOF-iceberg performance profiles based on individual strengths and limitations can be developed following the procedures proposed earlier for emotion profiling. Finally, the intensity of emotional reactions in soccer players is related to athletes' needs, attitudes and values. These aspects are the areas of social psychology and sociology that could also provide some insight into emotion.

Finally, all of the discussion so far has focused more on analytical aspects of emotion as a component of the psychobiosocial state. A more holistic description of performance-related states is warranted, especially to enhance self-regulation and interventions at the individual and team levels. For instance, several studies that are under way explore one such promising avenue as the IZOF–based metaphorical description of situational states in highly skilled soccer players, ice-hockey players, and track-and field athletes (14).

By the way of conclusion, it can be suggested the situational analysis of performance in elite soccer is a really promising area that awaits researchers form different sub-disciplines and with different backgrounds. In other words, future impact of sport science upon the practice of soccer will depend to a larger degree upon joint interdisciplinary and multidisciplinary efforts in both research and consultancy.

Summary

The main focus of this paper was on the individualized approach to emotion-performance relationships in skilled soccer players. Conceptual, methodological, and empirical aspects of this research direction and consultancy based on the Individual Zones of Optimal Functioning (IZOF) model was briefly described. Prediction and explanation of interactive effects of individually optimal and dysfunctional subjective emotional experiences upon athletic performance were proposed. Selective empirical findings testing the basic assumptions of the IZOF model in soccer were described and future research directions and practical implications were suggested.

References

1. Borg G.: A category scale with ratio properties for intermodal and interindividual comparisons. In: Geiss H.-G. Petzold P. (Eds.). *Psychophysical judgement and the process of perception,* pp.25-34, 1982.
2. Borg, G.: *Borg's Perceived exertion and pain scales.* Champaign, IL.: Human Kinetics, 1998
3. Bortoli, L., Robazza, C., & Nougier, V.: Emotion in hockey and rugby. In: *Proceedings of the 9th World Congress of Sport Psychology,* pp.136-138, 1997.
4. Hanin, Y.L.: Mezhlichnostnyje konflikty v sportivnykh igrakh (Interpersonal conflicts in soccer). *Teoria I Praktika Fiskultury,* 7, pp. 11-14, 1976.
5. Hanin, Y.L.: O srochnoi diagnostike sostojanija sportsmena v gruppe (On the express diagnostics of athletes state anxiety in the group). *Teoria I Praktika Fizkulturi,* **8**, 8-11, 1977.

6. Hanin, Y.: The state-trait anxiety research on sports in the USSR. In: C.D. Spielberger & R. Diaz-Guerrero (Eds.), *Cross-Cultural Anxiety.* Vol.**3**, pp. 45-64, 1986.

7. Hanin, Y.: Interpersonal and intragroup anxiety in sports. In: D. Hackfort & C.D. Spielberger (Eds.), *Anxiety in sports,* pp. 19–28, 1989.

8. Hanin, Y.L.: Individual Zones of Optimal Functioning (IZOF) model: An Idiographic Approach to Performance Anxiety. In: K. Henschen and W. Straub (Eds.). *Sport Psychology: An Analysis of Athlete Behavior,* pp. 103-119, 1995.

9. Hanin, Y. L.: Social Psychology and Sport: Communication Processes in Top Performance Teams. *Sport Science Review,* 1 (2), 13-28, 1992.

10. Hanin, Y.L.: Mental Preparation of soccer players for International Matches. In: *Collection of UEFA papers, Fourth Course for European Youth Coaches,* pp. 1-12, 1993.

11. Hanin, J.: Hyvä souoritus syntyy tunteella. (Good performance comes from emotions). *Jalkapallo Valmentaja (Football Coach),* 6, 18-19, 1994a.

12. Hanin, J.: Pelaajan Optimaalinen Työvire (Players' Optimal Working State). In: *SOK palloiluseminaari.* Muistio 10, 10-24, 1994b.

13. Hanin, Y. L.: Emotions and athletic performance: individual zones of optimal functioning (IZOF) model. *European Yearbook of Sport Psychology,* **1**, 29-72. 1997.

14. Hanin, Y.L.: Successful and poor performance and emotions. In: Hanin Y. L. (Ed.). *Emotions in Sport,* Champagin, IL.: Human Kinetics, 2000 (in press).

15. Hanin, Y.L., Syrjä, P.: Performance Affect in Soccer Players: An Application of the IZOF Model. *Intern J. Sports Med.* 16: 4: 264-269, 1995a.

16. Hanin, Y.L. & Syrjä, P.: Performance Affect in Junior Ice Hockey Players: An Application of the Individual Zones of Optimal Functioning Model. *The Sport Psychologist, 9, 169-187, 1995b.*

17. Hanin, Y.L. & Syrjä, P.: Predicted, actual and recalled Affect in Olympic-level soccer players: idiographic assessments on individualised scales. *Journal of Sport and Exercise Psychology,* 18: 325-335, 1996.

18. Martens, R., Vealey, R. S., & Burton, D.: *Competitive Anxiety in Sport,* Champaign, IL.: Human Kinetics, 1990.

19. Pesonen, T.: *Tunteiden yhteys suoritukseen juniorijalkapalloilijoilla.* (Emotion-performance relationship in junior soccer players). Unpublished Master's Thesis. Dept. Psychology, Jyväskylä University, Jyväskylä, Finland, 1995.

20. Smith, R.E., Smoll, F. L., & Schutz, R.W.: Measurement and correlates of sport-specific cognitive and somatic trait anxiety: The Sport Anxiety Scale. *Anxiety Research,* 2, 263-280, 1990.

21. Spielberger, C.D., Gorsuch, R.L., & Lushene, R.E.: Manual for the State-Trait Anxiety Inventory (STAI). Palo Alto, CA.: Consulting Psychologists Press, 1970.

22. Syrjä, P.: *Performance related emotions in highly skilled soccer players: A longitudinal study testing the IZOF model.* Ph.D. Thesis. Jyväskylä, Finland: Jyväskylä University Press, 1999 (in press).

23. Syrjä, P., & Hanin, Y.: Measurement of emotion in sport: a comparison of individualized and normative scales. In: Proceedings of the 9th *World Congress of Sport Psychology*. Part 2, pp. 682-684, 1997a.
24. Syrjä, P. & Hanin, Y.L.: Individualised and group-oriented measures of emotion in sport: a comparative study. In: Abstracts of the 2nd *Annual Congress of the European College of Sports Science,* pp. 641-642, 1997b.
25. Syrjä, P., Hanin, Y., & Pesonen, T.: Emotion and performance relationship in soccer players. In: *Proceedings of the 9th European Congress on Sport Psychology,* Part 1, pp. 191-197, 1995.
26. Watson, D. & Tellegen A.: Towards a consensual structure of mood. *Psychological Bulletin,* 98, 219-235, 1985.

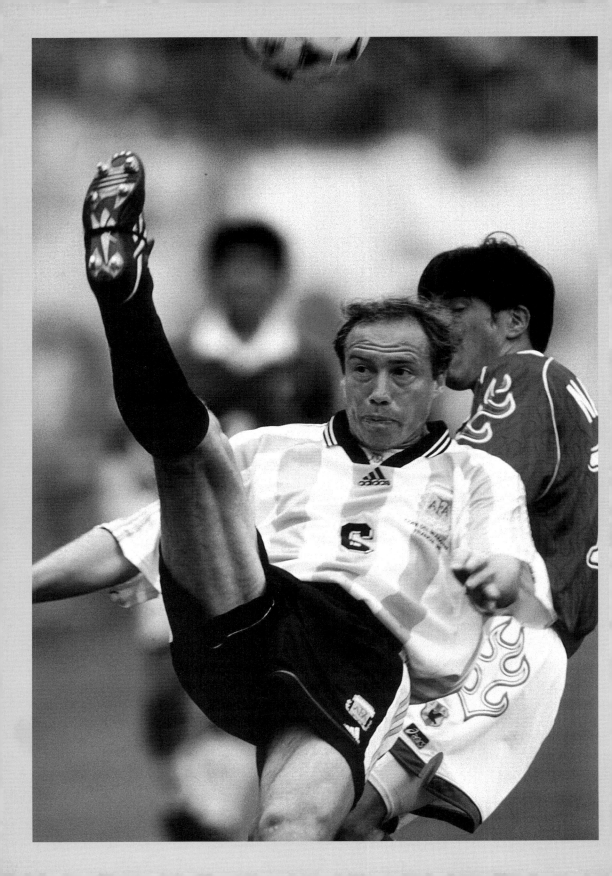

The physiological demands of soccer

Thomas Reilly

Synopsis

Match analysis can be used to provide a comprehensive picture of players' activities during a soccer game. Positional differences in work-rate profiles have been established. There are influences also of the style of play, the fitness of the competitors and their nutritional states. The physiological demands are largely aerobic but crucial aspects of play are supported by anaerobic processes. Skills of the game add to the energy costs of activity. These demands have consequences for the fitness of players, and for their weekly and seasonal training regimens.

Introduction

Soccer at a high standard engages a wide range of skills and abilities. The need to be able to control and pass a ball, kick and shoot with accuracy and power, win the ball in the air, execute tackles to perfection, dispossess opponents or dribble past them are some of the more obvious skills. The coach will recognise those players who demonstrate tactical "know-how", time their moves into space, evade opposing formations or create opportunities to win matches where there seemed to be none. Also important is the player's awareness of what is happening within the game, a sense of the configuration of one's team-mates and the lay-out of opponents, and above all anticipation of where the play is leading to – in other words, an ability to "read the game". These are some of the characteristics associated with soccer performance.

The contemporary elite male soccer player needs a foundation of systematic preparation in order to cope with the many demands that competitive matches impose on him and thereby display his artistry. This is particularly so at the professional level where gaps in fitness will be ruthlessly exposed by the opposition. It is in the preparation of players for the demands of the game that scientific principles can complement the expertise and judgement of the coach. This scientific support is only now being utilised by many of the top European professional teams. Nevertheless, it is reasonable to ask "what exactly are the physiological stresses and demands of soccer play and how in fact can they be measured?"

Match analysis

An indication of the demands of the game can be obtained by recording what players in fact do during the course of the game. This calls for objective, reliable and valid measures: video-recordings of one player at a time, followed by computerised tracking of his path (and actions) now fulfil these criteria. A significant data-base on the movements of individual players has been built up over the last 25 years in laboratories, such as the "science and football" facility at the Research Institute for Sport and Exercise Sciences (Liverpool John Moores University). This bank of information provides evidence that there has been a significant increase in the pace of play in the top English League over this time, although the speed-up did not become pronounced until about 1990. This coincided with the success of European club sides such as A.C. Milan whose players tended to play at a high tempo and put firm emphasis on all-round fitness.

The consensus of reports on top-level matches is that outfield players cover between 9 and 12 kilometres in a game. The majority of this is at submaximal or low intensity (walking, jogging, cruising), the ratio of low intensity (jogging, walking) to high intensity (sprints) events being 7:1 in terms of time. Strenuous efforts (cruising and sprinting) are called for every 30 seconds on average and all-out sprints averaging a distance of 15 metres are demanded every 90 seconds on average. Each game entails over 1000 discrete activities, a change in activity every 5-6 seconds and a pause of 3 seconds once every 2 minutes (16). The activity profiles are acyclical in that the discrete actions rarely follow a particular pattern: nevertheless they are reproducible from game to game when the whole-game profile is taken into account. The most consistent observation is in the high intensity activity which seems to differ very little between games (6).

The overall distance covered represents only a crude index of players' work-rate during competition. Critically important is the timing of runs to support team mates, to assume strategic positions for defensive or offensive actions, to maintain the required shape of the team's forma-tion and to entice opposing players out of position. This applies despite observations that less than 2% of the total distance covered is completed in possession of the ball. The exercise 'off-the-ball' incorporates accele-rations and decelerations, abrupt changes of direction, angled runs and movements backwards and sideways. Most importantly, they incor-porate actions directly involved in playing the ball and contesting pos-session.

Physiological Components of Soccer Work-Rates

The major part of activities during soccer are aerobic, consisting of submaximal exercise intensities. This is corroborated by the strong relationship found between maximal oxygen uptake and distance covered in a game (22). This relation is strengthened when 'fitness' is indicated by performance in an intermittent endurance exercise test and results are correlated with selected aspects of work-rate within the game (3). The more impressive aerobic fitness test profiles are shown by midfield players who tend also to cover the greater distances. In contrast, the lower distances among out-fielders are found in centre backs who cover an average of 20% less distance than the midfield players but tend to possess high anaerobic power (rather than high aerobic power) values. These comparisons are illustrated in Fig. 1, the positional differences being evident in observations of over 50 games. The variability (as evidenced by the size of the line bars on the top of the graphs) is greater in the full-backs, due to their greater flexibility than other roles.

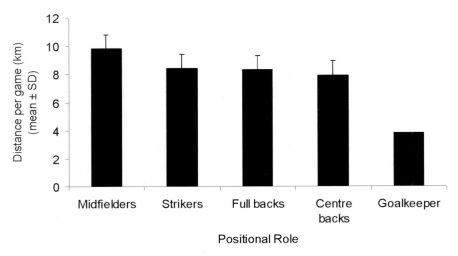

Fig. 1 The average (standard deviations are demonstrated by the lines) distance covered in top English league football according to positional role. These observations were first made in the 1970s but are still evident in the top leagues in the major European countries.

Anaerobic metabolism refers to the use of energy by muscles in the absence of an adequate oxygen supply, a function that can deliver high energy output but for a very brief period. Whilst the predominant activities may be aerobic in nature, critical events in the game are dependent on anaerobic efforts. Such anaerobic efforts usually require appropriate timing of movements (moving at exactly the right time), the execution of short quick movements (particularly by defenders and by forwards) to win the ball and agile movements to get past opponents. Important also is the ability to recover between bouts of exercise in order to be prepared for further all-out efforts when opportunities arise. In this respect a good aerobic fitness helps in the recovery from bouts of anaerobic exercise.

The work-rate profile shows a tendency to decline towards the end of a game (15). This is least pronounced in subjects with high aerobic fitness but is also linked with a fall in glycogen stores contained within the leg muscles. Saltin (26) showed that four players who started a game with below normal muscle glycogen levels (as a result of training hard the previous day) were affected more by fatigue than were the five players with normal muscle glycogen stores pre-match. The most evident feature of performance in the fatigued players was in a lower number of sprints 'off-the-ball'. Carbohydrates stored in the liver and in skeletal muscles both provide the muscles with fuel for exercise, but carbohydrate broken down in the liver also furnish the cells of the central nervous system with glucose, thereby providing the brain with its energy source. However, blood glucose tends to be high at the end of a game in most cases, with little evidence of hypoglycaemia occurring.

An increase in goals scored towards the end of the game is further evidence of fatigue at this time (17). Its explanation is likely to be accounted for by a complex of phenomena, including increased risk-taking by the team that is behind, a change in tactics due to the proximity of the end of the game, and lapses in concentration or mental fatigue.

Deterioration in mental performance related to soccer specific decision-making is evident only in less-skilled players (12). These trends have implications for the pacing of efforts throughout the game and also the nutritional strategies to last the entire 90 minutes of play. The strategies should embrace habitual dietary practices, nutritional preparation for competition, energy and fuel intake both during and following match-play.

The style of play will also influence the intensity of exercise during matches. The so-called "direct" method of play, pressurising opponents and moving the ball quickly into attack, increases the physiological demands on players. This approach has been adopted by teams in the English professional soccer leagues and by the Republic of Ireland and Norwegian national teams, for example. International matches in South America entail players covering about 1 kilometre less than the players in the English Premier League where a slow methodical build-up of attacks is not favoured (9). Man-to-man marking is also more demanding than zone coverage (11). Experience is that these styles have been modified to cope with environmental stresses, such as altitude at the 1986 World Cup in Mexico or the 1997 Copa America in Bolivia, and heat at the 1994 World Cup in the USA.

Of course there are additional activities besides movement around the pitch that imply direct involvement in the game. Centre-backs and strikers jump to head the ball 20 times a game on average, the corresponding figure being 11 for full-backs and 10 for midfield players. Tackles are completed at roughly the same rate, being greatest among defenders and least among the forwards (2). The success rate of all skills (passing, tackling and so on) decreases as play progresses up the field from defence into attack, highlighting the increased pressure on the player with the ball as the play approaches the opponents' goal (20).

Physiological investigations

Methods used in monitoring physiological responses to competition have been indirect or non-invasive and researchers have at least to some extent accepted the use of friendly or model games for this purpose. The key physiological issue is how much energy do players use in a match. Energy expenditures during match-play have been estimated from both work-rate profiles and heart-rate values (5, 16). The heart rates averaged throughout the game are then related to heart rate – oxygen consumption relationships determined for individual players in laboratory conditions. Alternative methods such as expired gas collections from Douglas bags or meteorological balloons worn on the back, or use of portable radio telemetry systems carried as a back-pack, to measure oxygen consumption are impractical in real games. Chemical techniques such as the doubly-labelled water method may prove useful in the future: these means require players to drink an isotopic solution and later provide urine or blood samples for the energy turn-over to be calculated. The overall outcome would be a clear picture of whether the player being monitored is in energy balance over a period of about a week and what the daily energy requirements to support both training and competition actually are.

Estimates are in general agreement that soccer competition at top level entails an energy expenditure of 4000-6000 kJ for a 70 kg player. This represents an average of about 70% of maximal oxygen uptake ($\dot{V}O_{2\,max}$) and is roughly approaching the rate at which a marathon runner competes. The active muscles are not the only organs needing a steady supply of energy from the bloodstream: the brain is integrally involved in soccer play (in continually making decisions and tactical choices), glucose being its sole source of energy. Blood glucose levels do not identify hypoglycaemia or the fall in blood glucose as a major problem for the team as a whole, although the variability reported for glucose levels at the end of a game indicate one or two individuals may suffer (4). It is likely that the repeated high-intensity bouts will reduce muscle and liver glycogen stores appreciably. This highlights the need to be adequately provided with carbohydrate before the game (i.e. the day before) and pay attention to restoring carbohydrate levels after the game (see page 117). Circulating fatty acids are raised by the end of the game in much the same way as they are elevated in endurance runners but deployment of protein metabolism is not pronounced. Wagenmakers *et al.* (27) demonstrated a contribution of branched chain amino acids towards metabolism over 90 min exercise at roughly the exercise intensity of soccer play, but its magnitude was calculated to be less than 5% of total fuel use. Consequently, the use of amino acids as energy supplements is not recommended for soccer players.

Blood lactate levels vary throughout the game and at times may reach levels in excess of 8 mM (10). Lactate is a product of anaerobic glycolysis and its appearance in blood represents the imbalance between production from within muscle and its clearance rate. It is thought that athletes can sustain exercise continuously up to a level corresponding to about 4 mM, known as lactate steady state. Breathing also begins to be challenged during exercise that is above this intensity. Soccer entails a variation of the exercise intensity on a non-systematic basis and lactate produced in the anaerobic efforts may be oxidised during the intervening recovery periods. Consequently lactate levels recorded at the end of the game are dependent on the activities of the previous 5 minutes (5). The lower blood lactate levels immediately post-match compared to observations at the end of the first half reflect both the increased proportional use of fat as a fuel for active muscles as the game progresses and the decline in intensity of effort as evidenced by the occurrence of fatigue. These factors should be taken into consideration when interpreting blood lactate levels during or after soccer matches.

Heart rates during match-play tend to average about 170 beats.min[-1]. The variability about this value is small. Heart rates may remain at this level towards the end of the game, despite a fall in work-rate. This may reflect the role of the circulatory system in regulating body temperature and preventing over-heating as well as transporting oxygen to the active muscles.

Work-rate profiles generally underestimate the energy requirements of the game. This is because the changes in velocity and skills of the game are not taken into account in a calculation of distances covered. Moving sideways or backwards increases energy expenditure and perceived exertion more than does normal locomotion (Fig. 2). Executing skills such as dribbling the ball also elevates energy expenditure

a

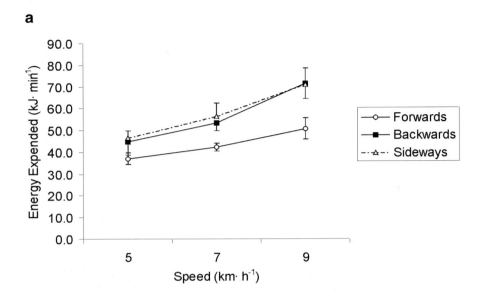

b

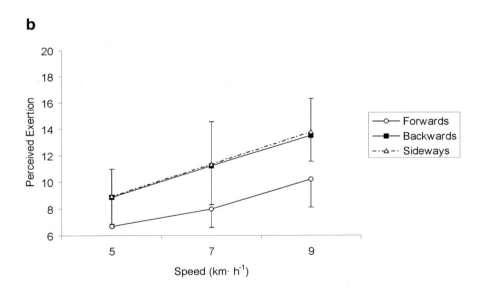

Fig. 2 The energy expended (measured in kilojoules per minute) at three different speeds of running forwards, backwards and sideways (a). The energy is elevated in the unorthodox movements compared to the natural forwards running. The corresponding ratings of perceived exertion are shown in (b). Data from 19.

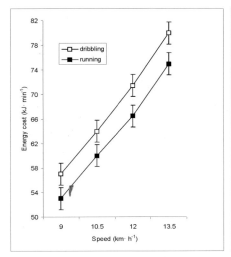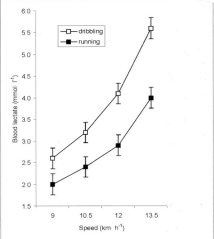

Fig. 3 The excess physiological cost of dribbling compared to normal running is evident in energy expenditure (left) and blood lactate (right) responses (n=8). Measurements are shown for 4 different speeds. Means ± SD are given. Data from 18.

and blood lactate more than does running at the same speed (Fig. 3). The implication is that these activities should be incorporated in training programmes where possible. A simple example is a progressive shuttle run where the player sprints from a scratch line to another 5, then 10, then 15, then 20 metres away, returning to the scratch line after each run, taking the ball with him and controlling it while he does so at speed.

Footballers' characteristics

The requirements for top soccer are many and varied, players needing the aerobic capabilities to sustain exercise for 90 (sometimes 120 minutes in cases of "extra-time"), the ability to accelerate quickly over short distances, decelerate or change direction without prior warning. Besides they must frequently generate high anaerobic power in jumping, tackling, shooting and so on. They need agility to cope with the changes in direction, muscle flexibility in stretching for a ball and strong connective tissue to withstand physical trauma. Their muscular make-up reflects the repetitive kicking and force-generating actions of the game. Players tend to have more skeletal muscle mass than normal and have a more muscular or 'mesomorphic' shape. They cannot afford to carry any extra depots of fat which would both slow them down and adversely affect jumping power (15). In this respect the footballer is unique, requiring a combination of different characteristics that are limiting factors in performance of other sports.

The physiological profiles of soccer players have been comprehensively reviewed by Reilly (15) and Bangsbo (5). A physiological profile of a team provides detail on the overall state of fitness of the squad. This may vary according to the physical training regimens employed, the frequency of competition, the stage of the competitive season, and so on. It can help in identifying strengths and weaknesses of individual players within the team. Physiological attributes may be depressed in players without adequate fitness training, on return to play after injury, and at times of overtraining.

The $\dot{V}O_{2\,max}$ of professional football players does improve significantly in the pre-season period when there is an emphasis on aerobic training (14). When two teams of equal skill meet, the one with superior aerobic fitness would have the edge, being able to play the game at a faster pace throughout. Apor (1) provided data on Hungarian players which showed perfect rank-order correlation between mean $\dot{V}O_{2\,max}$ of the team and finishing position in the Hungarian First Division championship. Mean $\dot{V}O_{2\,max}$ for the first, second, third and fifth teams were 66.6, 64.3, 63.3 and 58.1 ml kg^{-1} min^{-1}, respectively. Whilst these differences may appear small, it seems they are sufficient to have an impact on performance when the profile of the entire team is considered. Common factors such as stability in the team, avoidance of injury, and so on, help to maintain both $\dot{V}O_{2\,max}$, general fitness level and team performance independently.

The Weekly Regimen

Typically each week's training culminates in week-end competition. The weekly pattern is generally a build up to a mid-week peak and a tapering off in preparation for the match (24). The lull early in the week allows for recovery from the previous game and the aftermath of its physical contacts. A tapering is advised in view of the benefits of commencing each game with muscle glycogen levels replenished. This

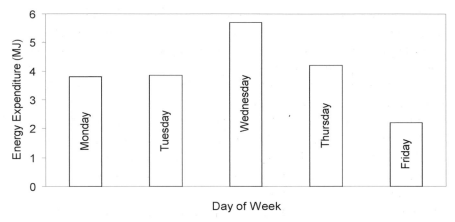

Fig. 4 The energy (MJ) expended in training by soccer players (average body mass = 73 ± 8 kg) in a typical week prior to a competitive match on Saturday (n=23). Mean values are given for each week-day.

preparation can be complemented by nutritional strategies to bias the players' diet towards carbohydrates (see page 117). The energy expended during training in a typical week in an England Premier League squad is illustrated in Fig. 4. Matches were on Saturday with no training on Sunday.

This model must be modified when two matches are scheduled in one week. In such events the training programme has to be curtailed in order that the players are not fatigued from training when they start the mid-week game. Nevertheless, the physical conditioning aspects of training cannot be shelved completely and there may be a need to focus on selective aspects of fitness in these short interim periods.

Time of day at which training is conducted is also a factor. Gross muscular performance tends to peak at about 18:00 hours when body temperature is at its daily high point (25). Common practice among professional teams is that training is planned for the morning whether matches are in the afternoon or in the evening. Training is conducted in the morning so as to control players' habitual activity more easily rather than for chronobiological reasons which consider the human's body clock. Whilst evidence would support skills acquisition sessions for morning time, strength training sessions are best executed in the late afternoon and evening when muscle strength reaches its day-time peak. This time of day would also help avoid risks of dehydration and hyperthermia in hot countries.

Recovery from matches

Soccer players frequently may have to play up to 3 games in 8 days, notably if engaged in European club competitions in mid-week and in their own national leagues at week-ends. At times of congested fixture lists they may be required to play 2 games within 3 days. In such instances it is imperative to adopt strategies which optimise recovery between matches.

Immediately post-game an active low-intensity warm down accelerates recovery processes (21). Whilst warm down procedures are readily adopted in many sports, they are not yet part of the soccer playing culture. Players may also have reduced glycogen stores in their leg muscles at the end of a match. It is important that the restoration of carbohydrate stores is commenced in the first 2 hours of finishing a game as glycogen resynthesis can be accelerated at this time. Fluid replacement is also urgent since players may lose 2-3 hours in sweat in the course of a game. Energy and electrolyte drinks offer the best combination and can be complemented by making solid carbohydrate food available (13). The regeneration can be continued with a high carbohydrate breakfast the next day. Up to 600 g of carbohydrate should be ingested the day following a match, though this quantity might be exceeded in players with a high work-rate or a large body mass.

Light training at submaximal intensities can be performed the day following a match. Delayed onset muscle soreness generally peaks 48 hours following exercise which entails repetitive stretch-shortening cycle movements. These actions occur in soccer in stretching to tackle, decelerate, kick and in other contexts. Training regimens incorporating 'stretch-shortening cycle' exercise are know as plyometrics. Plyometric training especially during the pre-season phase offers protection for 3 weeks or more against this form of muscle soreness (7). The so-called 'delayed onset muscle soreness' associated with eccentric actions doesn't seem to be a major problem with soccer players who are well conditioned. Nevertheless, strenuous plyometric drills should be avoided in between matches that quickly follow one another so that 'delayed onset muscle soreness' is not accentuated.

Deep water training provides one method of maintaining fitness during an intense period of competition. The method appears to be effective in aiding rehabilitation and as subjects can attain about 70%

$\dot{V}O_{2\,max}$ when running in deep water, would provide a strong stimulus in days of recovering from match stresses (8). One particular advantage is that impact loading is reduced. This method has potential for clubs with access to swimming pool facilities.

Seasonal Variations in Training

The more intense training regimens tend to be employed in the pre-season conditioning of players. This is largely due to the need to counteract the detraining effects that accrue between competitive seasons. Players who maintain a low intensity programme during the off-season manage to retain aerobic and muscular fitness relatively well in addition to controlling their body weight.

Pre-season conditioning programmes tend to emphasise endurance and aerobic fitness at the expense of muscular strength. Consequently players may commence the competitive period with suboptimal muscle strength and therefore an increased risk of injury due to muscle weakness (23). The tendency can be corrected by incorporating a balance of training stimuli in the pre-season training. During the competitive season players may frequently have to compete twice in one week. In such an event a considerable training stimulus is provided by playing the game. Once mid-season is reached a primary objective should be to maintain the fitness level already acquired to the end of the competitive season. This does not necessarily apply to the whole team, since some players may require additional training in cases of returning to the squad following injury, for example.

Overview

Physiological investigations have increased our understanding of the stresses associated with playing the game of soccer. The intensity of exercise during elite play has placed aerobic fitness as a major requirement, although anaerobic efforts are emphasised during direct involvement in play. The physiological demands vary with positional role, styles of play and environmental circumstances. Cultural and national factors, independent of these also influence the pace at which matches are played.

References

1. Apor, P. Successful formulae for fitness training. In: *Science and Football* (eds. T. Reilly, A. Lees, K. Davids and W. Murphy). London: E. and F.N. Spon, pp. 95-107, 1988.
2. Bangsbo, J. The physiology of soccer – with special reference to intermittent exercise. *Acta Physiologia Scandinavica,* 151 Suppl. 619, 1994.
3. Bangsbo, J. The energy demands in competitive soccer. *Journal of Sports Sciences,* 12, p. 5-12, 1994a.
4. Bangsbo, J. Physiological demands. In: *Football (Soccer)* (ed. B. Ekblom). London: Blackwell, pp. 43-58, 1994b.
5. Bangsbo, J. The physiological profile of soccer players. *Sports Exercise and Injury,* 4, 144-150, 1998.
6. Bangsbo, J., Norregaard, L. and Thorsoe, F. Activity profile by competition soccer. *Canadian Journal of Sports Sciences,* 16, 110-116, 1991.
7. Cleak, M.M. and Eston, K. G. Delayed onset muscle soreness: mechanisms and management. *Journal of Sports Sciences,* 10, 325-341, 1992.
8. Dowzer, C. and Reilly, T. (1998). Deep water running. *Sports Exercise and Injury,* 4, 56-61, 1998.
9. Drust, B., Reilly, T. and Rienzi, E. Analysis of work-rate in soccer. *Sports Exercise and Injury,* 4, 151-155, 1998.
10. Ekblom, B. Applied physiology in soccer. *Sports Medicine,* 3, 50-60, 1986.
11. Gerisch, G., Rutemoller, E. and Weber, K. Sportsmedical measurements of performance in soccer. In: *Science and Football* (eds T. Reilly, A. Lees, K. Davids and W. Murph). London: E. and F.N. Spon, pp. 95-107, 1988.
12. Marriott, J., Reilly, T. and Miles, A. The effect of physiological stress on cognitive performance in a simulation of soccer. In: *Science and Football* (eds T. Reilly, J. Clarys and A. Stibbe), London: E. & F.N. Spon, pp. 261-264, 1993.
13. Maughan, R. J. and Leiper, J. B. Fluid replacement requirements in soccer. *Journal of Sports Sciences,* 12, S29-34, 1994.
14. Reilly, T. *What research tells the coach about soccer.* Aahperd: Washington. 1979.
15. Reilly, T. Motion characteristics. In: *Football (Soccer)* (ed. B. Ekblom). London: Blackwell, pp. 31-42, 1994.
16. Reilly, T. Motion analysis and physiological demands. In: *Science and Soccer* (ed. T. Reilly). London: E. and F.N. Spon, pp. 65-81, 1996.
17. Reilly, T. Energetics of high-intensity exercise (soccer) with particular reference to fatigue. *Journal of Sports Sciences,* 15, 257-263, 1997.
18. Reilly, T. and Ball, D. The physiological cost of dribbling a soccer ball. *Research Quarterly for Exercise and Sport,* 55, 267-271, 1984.
19. Reilly, T. and Bowen, T. Exertional costs of changes in directional modes of running. *Perceptual and Motor Skills,* 58, 49-50, 1984.
20. Reilly, T. and Holmes, M. A preliminary analysis of selected soccer skills. *Physical Education Review,* 6, 64-71, 1983.

21. Reilly, T. and Rigby, M. Effect of warm-down on recovery from soccer. *Communication to the Fourth World Congress on Science and Football* (Sydney, Australia), February 22-26, 1999.

22. Reilly, T. and Thomas, V. An analysis of work-rate in different positional roles in professional football match-play. *Journal of Human Movement Studies,* **2**, 87-98, 1976.

23. Reilly, T. and Thomas, V. Effects of a programme of pre-season training on the fitness of soccer players. *Journal of Sports Medicine and Physical Fitness,* 17, 401-412, 1977.

24. Reilly, T. and Thomas, V. Estimated energy expenditure of professional association footballers. *Ergonomics,* 22, 541-548, 1979.

25. Reilly, T., Atkinson, G. and Waterhouse, J. *Biological Rhythms and Exercise.* Oxford: Oxford University Press. 1997.

26. Saltin, B. Metabolic fundamentals in exercise. *Medicine and Science in Sports,* 5, 137-146, 1973.

27. Wagenmakers, A.J.M., Brookes, J.M. Coakley, J.H., Reilly, T. and Edwards, R.H.T. Exercise induced activation of the branched chain 2-oxo acid dehydrogenase in human muscle. *European Journal of Applied Physiology,* 59, 159-167, 1989.

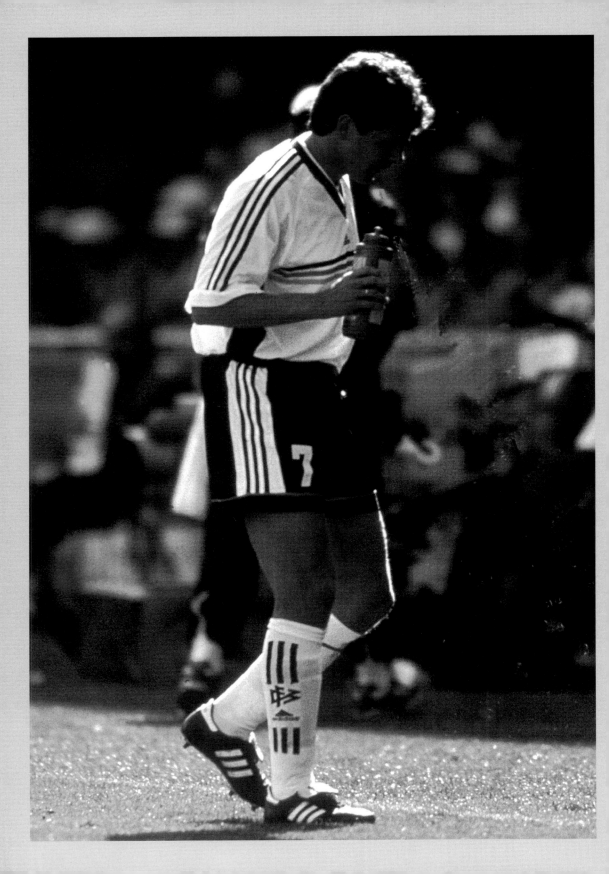

Nutrition in Soccer

Jens Bangsbo

Synopsis

In soccer the players perform high intense intermittent exercise for a long duration and the total energy cost of a game can be high. Muscle glycogen is the most important substrate and even a partial depletion of the muscle glycogen stores may limit performance. To fulfil the requirement of training and matches soccer players should have a balanced diet that contains large amounts of carbohydrate. In general it is important for the players to be conscious of the nutritive value of the food that they consume. In soccer the loss of body water, mainly due to the evaporation of sweat, can be more than three litres during competition. It is important for the players to take in fluid during a game and also during a training session to maintain the efficiency of the training. Besides reducing the net loss of body water, the intake of fluid can supply the body with carbohydrates.

Introduction

In determining proper nutritional recommendations in soccer, it is important to assess the requirements of soccer and determine whether substrate availability may limit performance. In soccer the intensity can alternate at any time and range from standing still to sprinting (Fig. 1). This is in contrast to sports disciplines like a 400-m and a marathon run in which during the entire event continuous exercise is

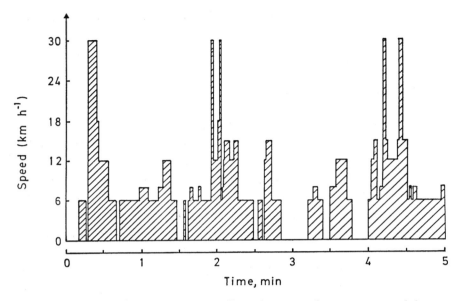

Fig. 1 An example of exercise intensities for a player in a five-minute period during a soccer match. Data from 5.

performed at a very high or at a moderate intensity, respectively. Due to the intermittent nature of soccer performance may not only be impaired toward the end of a match, but also after periods of intense exercise. Both types of fatigue might be related to the metabolic processes that occur during match play. Therefore, before discussing the diet of soccer players, energy provision and substrate utilisation during intermittent exercise and in soccer will be considered.

Energy production and Substrate utilisation in team sports

In soccer the exercise performed is intermittent. It is therefore important to know how metabolism and performance during an exercise bout are influenced by previous exercise. Through the years this has been investigated systematically by changing one of the variables at a time. Such studies form the basis for understanding the physiology of intermittent exercise. It has to be recognised that in most laboratory studies the variations in exercise intensity and duration are regular, whereas in many intermittent sports the changes in exercise intensity are irregular and can be almost random.

Anaerobic energy production

In a study subjects performed intermittent cycle exercise for 1 hour alternating between 15 s rest and 15 s of exercise at a work rate that for continuous cycling demanded maximum oxygen uptake (13). Considerable fluctuations in adenosinetriphosphate (ATP) and creatine phosphate (CP) occurred. The CP concentration after an exercise period was 40% of the resting level, and it increased to about 70% of the initial level in the subsequent 15 s recovery period, whereas the increase in muscle lactate was low.

Also in soccer, the CP concentration probably alternates continuously as a result of the intermittent nature of the game. Fig. 2 shows an example of the fluctuations of CP determined by nuclear magnetic resonance (NMR) during three 2-min intermittent exercise periods that each included short maximal contractions, low intensity contractions and rest. A pronounced decrease of CP was observed during the maximal contractions, but it almost reached pre-exercise value at the end of each 2-min intermittent contraction period (Fig. 2). Thus, although the net utilisation of CP is quantitatively small during competition, CP has a very important function as an energy buffer, providing phosphate for the resynthesis of ATP reaction during rapid elevations in the exercise intensity and the availability of CP may determine performance during some intense periods of a game.

Lactate in the blood taken during match play may reflect, but underestimate, the lactate production in a short period prior to the sampling (5). Thus, the concentration of lactate in the blood is often used as an indicator of the anaerobic lactacid energy production in sports. In soccer high lactate concentrations are often found suggesting that lactate production during a match can be very high.

Aerobic energy production

Heart rate determinations during match play can give an indication of to what extent the aerobic energy system is taxed. In soccer it has

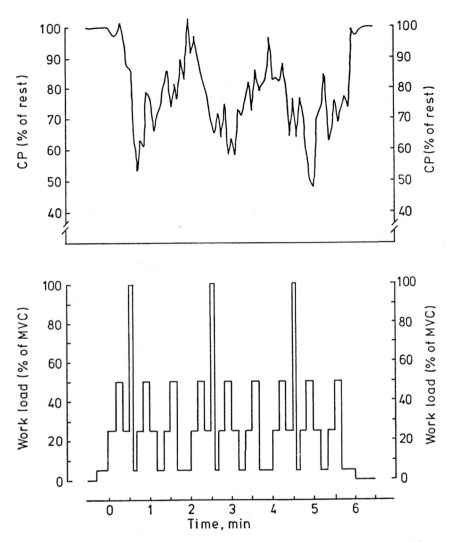

Fig. 2 Creatine phosphate (CP) concentration in m. gastrocnemius determined by nuclear magnetic resonance (upper panel) during isometric contractions with the calf muscles at alternating work loads (lower panel). The exercise consisted of three identical 2 min contraction periods, each including a maximal contraction. Data from 5.

been estimated that the aerobic energy production is around 70% of maximum oxygen uptake although the players are standing or walking for more than one-third of the game (5). One explanation of the high aerobic energy utilisation is that oxygen uptake in the recovery periods is high preceding intense exercise periods (5).

Substrate utilisation

The large aerobic energy production and the pronounced anaerobic energy turnover during periods of a match in soccer are associated with a large consumption of substrates. The dominant substrates are carbohydrate (CHO) and fat either stored within the exercising muscle or delivered via the blood to the muscles.

The carbohydrate used during a match is mainly the glycogen stored within the exercising muscles, but glucose extracted from the blood may also be utilised by the muscles. Information about the use of muscle glycogen during a match can be obtained from determinations of glycogen in muscle samples taken before and after the match. The difference in glycogen content represents the net utilisation of muscle glycogen, but it does not show the total glycogen turnover, since resynthesis of glycogen probably occurs during the rest and low intensity exercise periods during a match (5, 27). Muscle glycogen utilisation may be high in soccer. As an example, in a study of Swedish soccer players the average thigh muscle glycogen concentrations of five players were 96, 32 and 9 mmol•kg^{-1} w.w. before, at half time and after a non-competitive match, respectively (31). An important aspect to consider in soccer is that even though the muscle glycogen stores are not depleted the level of muscle glycogen may be limiting for performance (see below).

Fat oxidation is probably high during a soccer match. Studies focusing on recovery from intense exercise and intermittent exercise suggest that fat to a get extent is oxidised after intense exercise (7, 16). The primary source of the fat oxidised in the rest periods in between the exercises may be muscle or blood delivered triacylglycerol (7).

The role of protein metabolism in soccer is unclear, but studies with continuous exercise at a mean work rate and duration similar to soccer have shown that oxidation of proteins may contribute, but less than 10% of the total energy production (33).

Summary

In soccer the players perform high intense intermittent exercise, at times for a long duration. The intense exercise periods requires a high rate of energy turnover and the total energy cost of a game can be

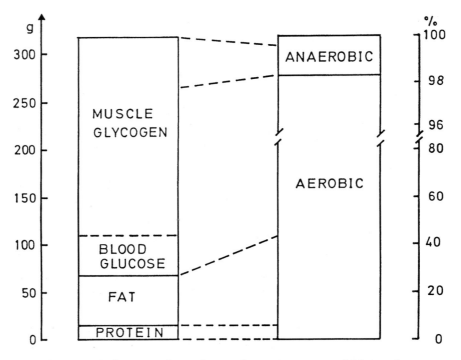

Fig. 3 Estimated relative aerobic and anaerobic energy turnover (right) and corresponding substrate utilization (left) during a soccer match. From 5.

high. Muscle glycogen appears to the most important substrate as is clear from Fig. 3, which shows an estimation of substrate utilisation during a soccer game. In soccer even a partial depletion of the muscle glycogen stores may limit performance. It should be noted that large inter-individual differences exist in the energy production during a match due to the variety of factors influencing the exercise intensity of a player, e.g. motivation, physical capacity and tactical role.

Diet in soccer

In this section the importance of nutrition in soccer is discussed and dietary recommendations to accommodate nutritional requirements for training and matches are provided. It should be emphasised that maintaining an adequate diet will improve the potential to reach a maximum level of performance, but does not ensure good performance during a match. There are many other factors that influence performance like technical abilities and tactical understanding.

Diet and performance in intermittent exercise

It is well established that performance during long-term continuous exercise is improved by intake of a carbohydrate rich diet in the days before the exercise. In order to evaluate whether a diet high in carbohydrates also affects performance during prolonged intermittent exercise, a study on eight professional Danish players was performed.

A soccer-specific intermittent exercise test was used to evaluate performance (Fig. 4). The players ran intermittently until they were exhausted and the test result was the total distance covered. The mean exercise intensity during the tests was 70-80% of maximum oxygen uptake, which resembles the average intensity during soccer.

The players performed the test on two occasions separated by 14 days. On one of the occasions the test was carried out with the players having ingested a diet containing 39% (Control-diet; C-diet) carbohydrates during the days before the test, and on the other occasion the players performed the test having consumed a high-carbohydrate diet (65% carbohydrate; CHO-diet) prior to the test. Both tests were carried out three days after a competitive soccer match with the diets maintained during the two days following the match. The order of the tests was assigned randomly. The total running distance of 17.1 km after the CHO-diet was significantly longer (0.9 km) than after the C-diet. Thus, increasing the CHO content in the diet from 39% or 355 g to 65% or 602 g per day (4.6 and 7.9 g per kg body mass) improved intermittent endurance performance. Similarly, it has been observed that performance during long-term intermittent exercise consisting of 6 s work periods separated by 30 s rest periods was related to the initial muscle glycogen concentration (2).

The findings in the above mentioned studies suggest that elevated muscle glycogen levels prior to competition do increase the mean work rate during a soccer match. In agreement with this suggestion, it was observed that the use of glycogen was more pronounced in the first compared to the second half of a game (31). Furthermore, the players with initially low glycogen covered a shorter distance and sprinted significantly less, particularly in the second half, than the players with

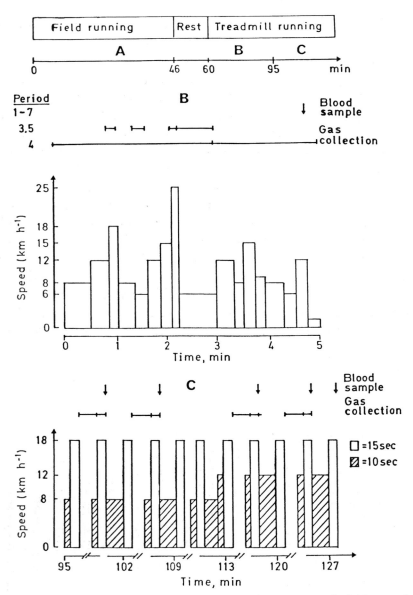

Fig. 4 Protocol of an intermittent endurance test. The test consisted of 46 min of intermittent field running (A) followed by 14 min of rest and then by two parts of intermittent treadmill running to exhaustion (B and C; upper panel). Middle panel shows part B of the treadmill running which consisted of seven identical 5-min intermittent exercise periods. Lower panel shows part C in which treadmill speed was alternated between 8 and 18 km·h⁻¹ for 10 and 15 s, respectively. After 17 min of part C the lower speed was elevated to 12 km·h⁻¹, and the running was continued until exhaustion. From 9.

normal muscle glycogen levels prior to a match (31). It can be assumed that the players would have been better prepared for the second half if the muscle glycogen stores had been higher prior to the match.

It may not only be towards the end of a match that the levels of muscle glycogen is affecting performance. In a study using 15 repeated 6 s sprints separated by 30 s rest periods it was found that performance was significantly increased when the subjects had elevated the muscle glycogen stores prior to the exercise (Fig. 5). In agreement with this findings it has been observed that high muscle glycogen levels did not affect performance in single intense exercise periods, but when exercise was repeated 1 h later fatigue occurred at a later stage when the subjects started with superior muscle glycogen concentrations (8). It is worthwhile to note that in both studies the muscle glycogen level was still high at the point of fatigue defined as an inability to maintain the required power output. During intense intermittent exercise both slow twitch (ST) and fast twitch (FT) fibres are involved (17) and a partial depletion of glycogen in some fibres, particular the FT-fibres, may result in a reduction in performance. These studies demonstrate that if

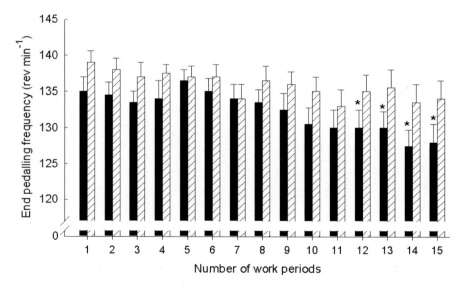

Fig. 5 Pedalling frequency during last 2 s of 15 6-s periods of intense cycling separated by 30 s rest periods with a diet low (filled bars) and high (hatched bars) in carbohydrates in the days before the test. The subjects were supposed to maintain a pedalling frequency of 140 revolutions per min. Note that after the high carbohydrate diet the subjects were better able to keep a high pedalling frequency. Data from 2.

the muscle glycogen levels are not high prior to a game performance of repeated intense exercise during the game may be impaired.

Diets of soccer players

The above mentioned studies clearly show that high glycogen levels are essential to optimise performance during intense intermittent exercise. However, soccer players may not actually consume sufficient amounts of carbohydrate, as illustrated in a study of Swedish elite soccer players. After a competitive match played on a Sunday, the players were monitored until the following Wednesday when they played a European Cup match. One light training session was performed on the Tuesday. Immediately after the match on Sunday, and on the following two days, muscle samples were taken from a quadriceps muscle

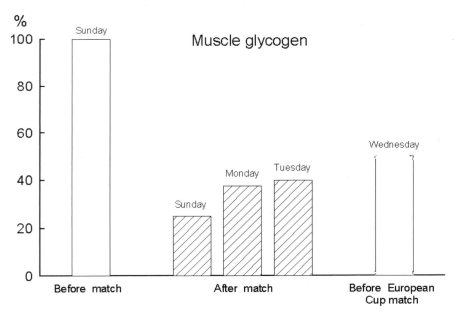

Fig. 6 The muscle glycogen content of a quadriceps muscle for players in a Swedish top-class soccer team, before and just after a league match (Sunday). The figure also gives muscle glycogen values at 24 and 48 hours after the match, and an estimate of the level before a European Cup match on the following Wednesday (dotted bar). The values are expressed in relation to the level before the league match (100%). Note that muscle glycogen was only restored to about 50% of "normal level" before the European Cup match. From 6.

for determination of glycogen content (Fig. 6). After the match the muscle glycogen content was found to be reduced to approximately 25% of the level before the match. Twenty-four hours (Monday) and forty-eight hours (Tuesday) later, the glycogen stores had only increased to 37% and 39% of the pre-match level, respectively. Muscle samples were not taken on the Wednesday because of the European Cup match, but it can be assumed that the glycogen stores were less than 50% of the pre-match levels. Thus, the players started the match with only about half of their normal muscle glycogen stores, which most likely reduced their physical performance potential.

The food intake of each player was on a separate occasion analysed during the same period (Sunday - Wednesday). The average energy intake per day was 20.7 MJ (approximately 4700 kcal), with a variation between players from 10.5 to 26.8 MJ. By use of the activity profile and body weight of each player, it was calculated that most of the players should have had an intake of at least 20 MJ. Therefore, for some of the players the total energy consumption was much lower than required.

The quality of the diet must also be considered, e.g. the proportion of protein, fat, and carbohydrate. The players' diet contained on average 14% protein of total energy intake (which lies within the recommended range), 47% carbohydrate and 39% fat. If these percentages are compared with those recommended of at least 60% carbohydrate and no more than 25% fat, it is evident that the carbohydrate intake by the players was too low on the days before the European Cup match. This factor, together with the relatively low total energy consumption of some players after the Sunday match, can explain the low muscle glycogen stores found on the days prior to the European Cup match. Thus, the diet of the players was inadequate for optimal physical performance.

It is clear that many soccer players are not aware of the importance of consuming large amounts of carbohydrates in the diet. It may be possible to achieve major changes in dietary habits just by giving the players appropriate information and advice. In the study concerning the effect of a carbohydrate rich diet on intermittent exercise performance, 60% of the soccer players' diet was controlled, whereas they within given guidelines could select the remaining 40% themselves. Using this procedure the average carbohydrate intake was increased from about 45% in the normal diet to 65% in the high-carbohydrate diet. The foods that were consumed in the carbohydrate rich diet are found in most households. This means it is not necessary to drastically change dietary habits in order to obtain a more appropriate diet.

Everyday diet

Carbohydrates

It is evident that eating a carbohydrate rich diet on the days before a match is of importance for performance. To consume a significant amount of carbohydrate in the everyday diet is also beneficial to meet

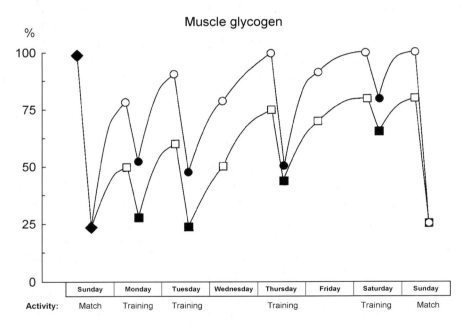

Fig. 7 The figure depicts a hypothetical example of how muscle glycogen stores can vary during a week for a soccer player with a high carbohydrate and a "normal" diet. There is a match on Sunday, a light training session on Monday, an intensive training session on Tuesday and Thursday, and a light training session Saturday. The filled symbols indicate the values after the match and training. Note that the glycogen stores are replenished at a faster rate with the high-carbohydrate diet, thus allowing for proper preparation for training and the subsequent match. In contrast, consuming a "normal" diet may result in reduced training efficiency and the glycogen stores may be lowered before the match. From 6.

the demands of training. Fig. 7 illustrates how the muscle glycogen stores may vary during a week of training for a player that consumed either a high-carbohydrate diet or a "normal" diet. During training some of the glycogen is used, and between training sessions the stores are slowly replenished. If the diet contains large amounts of carbohydrate it is possible to restore glycogen throughout the week. This may not be achieved if the diet is low in carbohydrates. An increase in glycogen storage is followed by an enhanced binding of water (2.7 g water per g glycogen). Thus, a high carbohydrate diet is likely to result in an increase in body weight, which might adversely affect performance in the early stage of the match. However, this effect is probably small and the benefit of high muscle glycogen concentrations before a match will probably outweigh the disadvantages of any increase in body weight. The maximal additional muscle glycogen synthesis when consuming a high CHO diet as compared with normal diet should be 150 g, which corresponds to a weight gain of less than 0.5 kg. Furthermore, a more pronounced breakdown of glycogen will enhance the release of water, which will reduce the net loss of water.

Protein

Protein is used primarily for maintaining and building up tissues, such as muscles. The amount of protein required in the diet is a topic frequently discussed, particularly with respect to those sports where muscle strength is important or where muscle injuries often occur. Soccer can be included in these categories. However, in most cases the players take in sufficient amount of proteins. For example, the daily intake of protein by Swedish and Danish soccer players were 2-3 grams per kilogram of body weight (9, 23), which is above the recommended daily intake for athletes of 1-2 grams per kilogram. In general, supplementing protein intake by tablets or protein powders is unnecessary for soccer players, even during an intensive strength training period.

Fat

Fat exists in two forms – saturated fat and unsaturated fat. The saturated fats are solid at room temperature (butter, margarine, and fat in meat) while unsaturated fats are liquid or soft at room temperature (vegetable oil, vegetable margarine, and fat in fish). Intake of unsaturated fats is essential for the body, and in contrast to saturated fats, unsaturated fats may aid in lowering the amount of cholesterol in the blood, thereby reducing the risk of heart disease. Therefore, it is important that saturated fats are replaced with unsaturated fats where possible. The total content of fat in the average diet of a soccer player is often too high and a general lowering of fat intake is advisable. One way of lowering the fat contain of the food is by reducing the intake of meat.

Minerals and vitamins

Food and drink supplies the body with fluids, energy-producing substrates, and other important components, such as salt, minerals, and vitamins. In a well-balanced diet most nutrients are supplied in sufficient amounts. However, there can be some exceptions.

Iron is an important element in haemoglobin, which binds to the red blood cells and aids in the transport of oxygen throughout the body. Therefore, an adequate iron intake is essential for athletes and especially for female soccer players, who lose blood and, thus, haemoglobin during menstruation. The recommended daily intake of iron for a player is approximately 20 milligrams, which should be ingested via solid foods rather than in tablet form, as iron found in solid foods is more effectively absorbed from the intestine to the blood. Animal organs (liver, heart, and kidneys), dried fruits, bread, nuts, strawberries and legumes are foods with a high content of iron. The most efficient way to promote iron absorption is by eating animal organs together with vitamin C from solid foods. It is advisable to increase iron intake in periods when players are expected to increase their red blood cell production, e.g. during the pre-season or when training at a high altitude.

A question commonly asked is whether or not players should supplement their diet with vitamins. In general, vitamin supplementation is not necessary, but there are conditions where it might be beneficial. For example, it is advisable to enhance vitamin E intake when training at high altitudes, and to use vitamin C and multiple B-vitamin supplements in hot climates.

Creatine

In soccer the rate of muscle CP utilisation is high during periods of match play and in the following recovery periods CP is resynthesized (see above). This leads to the question whether a soccer player can benefit from ingestion of creatine in a period before a match, as it has been shown that intake of creatine increase the CP and particularly creatine levels in muscles (20). For example, it was found that five subjects increased their total muscle creatine level (CP and creatine) by 25% after a creatine intake of 20 g•day[-1] for five days (19). An elevated level of creatine and CP may affect CP resynthesis after exercise (19), which may have an impact on the ability to perform intermittent exercise. In a study subjects performed ten 6-s high intensity exercise bouts on a cycle-ergometer separated by 24 s of rest, after they had ingested either creatine (20 g•day[-1]) or placebo for a week (3). The group which ingested creatine had a lower reduction in performance as the test progressed than the placebo-group. On the other hand, as one would expect, creatine ingestion appears to have no effect on prolonged (>10 min) continuous exercise performance (4).

Although creatine ingestion increases muscle CP and creatine concentration, it is doubtful that soccer players, except probably for vegetarians, will benefit from creatine supplementation, since creatine ingestion also causes an increases in body mass. It is still unclear what causes this increase, but it is most likely due to an increased accumulation of water. Nevertheless, a gain in body weight has a negative influence in sports in which the athletes have to move their body mass against gravity. For example, no difference in performance during intense intermittent running (Yo-Yo intermittent recovery test) was observed when a group of subjects performed the test after 7 days of creatine intake (20 g•day[-1]) compared to a test under control conditions. Furthermore, it is unclear how ingesting creatine for a period influences the body's own production of creatine and the enzymes that are related to creatine/CP synthesis and breakdown. It may be that a soccer player through regularly intake of creatine reduces his ability to produce CP and creatine, which may result in a reduction in the CP and creatine levels, when the player no longer is ingesting creatine. In addition, very little is known about any possible side effect of a frequent intake of creatine. High concentrations of creatine may have negative effects on the kidney, which has to eliminate the excess creatine as creatinine. One should also consider that ingestion of creatine could be seen as doping eventhough it is not on the IOC doping list. It may be argued that creatine is a natural compound and that it is contained in the food. However, it is almost impossible to get doses (10-20 g per day) of creatine corresponding to those used in the experiments which showed enhanced performance, as the content of creatine in 1 kg of raw meat is around 5 g.

Pre-training and pre-competition meal

On the day of a match the intake of fat and protein (especially derived from meat) should be restricted. The pre-training or pre-match meal should be ingested 3-4 hours prior to competition or training. If too much food is ingested after this time, there still may be undigested food in the stomach and intestine when the training or match begins. The meal should mainly contain a high amount of CHO. It has been demonstrated that ingestion of 312 g of CHO four hours prior to strenuous continuous exercise resulted in a 15% improvement in exercise performance, but no improvement was observed when either 45 or 156 g of CHO was ingested (32). A snack high in carbohydrate, e.g. bread with jam, may be eaten about 1.5 hours before the match. However, these time references are only guidelines. There are great individual differences in the ability to digest food. It is a good idea for players to experiment with a variety of foods at different times before training sessions.

An improvement in exercise performance has been observed if CHO was ingested immediately before exercise (26). On the other hand, glucose ingestion 30-60 min prior to severe exercise has been shown to produce a rapid fall in blood glucose with the onset of exercise, an increase in muscle glycogen utilisation and a reduction in exercise time to exhaustion (13). However, not all studies have shown a detrimental effect of ingesting CHO before exercise, and some studies have shown improved performance after CHO ingestion in the last hour prior to strenuous exercise (18). The differences seem to be closely related to the glucose and insulin responses. When exercising with a high insulin concentration there is an abnormally large loss of glucose from the blood resulting in a low blood glucose concentration. Consequently, the muscles and the brain gradually become starved of glucose, which eventually leads to fatigue.

Food intake after exercise

Physical activity is a powerful stimulus to glycogen resynthesis as was elegantly shown in a study, where a glycogen depleted leg attained muscle glycogen levels twice as high as the resting control leg during a three day period (10). In addition, it seems that the muscles are particularly sensitive to glucose uptake and glycogen resynthesis in the period immediately after exercise (29, 21). It was found that the rate of glycogen resynthesis during the first two hours after CHO intake was faster if CHO was ingested immediately following an exercise bout, rather than delaying the intake by two hours (21). It has been suggested that there is an upper limit of carbohydrate ingested, which can be used for glycogen synthesis. Ivy et al. (22) found the same increase in muscle glycogen storage after exercise with a diet containing 1.5 g or 3.0 g per kg b.w. In addition, the actual number of meals ingested appears not to influence the rate of glycogen resynthesis (14). On the other hand, is has been observed that the rate of glycogen rebuilding could be further elevated by very frequent ingestion of liquid carbohydrate (17).

It has also been demonstrated, that the increase in muscle glycogen was larger during the first 6 h after exercise when a diet containing simple carbohydrates was consumed compared with a diet consisting of complex carbohydrates (24). Furthermore, glucose and sucrose result in a faster muscle glycogen synthesis than fructose, which might be of more benefit in the restoration of liver glycogen (11). Nevertheless, the muscle glycogen stores can reach resting levels 20 h after exercise, with both a simple and a complex CHO diet if the total CHO content is great enough (24). Thus, unless the players train or play within 24 h, the type of carbohydrates ingested seems unimportant. An inverse relationship between the rate of glycogen rebuilding and the muscle glycogen concentration after prolonged continuous exercise or soccer match play has been demonstrated (23, 28). Therefore, it appears that every player can replenish the muscle glycogen stores within 24 hrs after a match, irrespective of the magnitude of the decrease of carbohydrates during the game. However, other factors have been shown to influence the rate of glycogen synthesis. Glycogen restoration was impaired after exhaustive running that produced muscle damage (11), and similar findings were obtained after eccentric exercise (34). In one study the muscle glycogen level ten days after a 45 min exercise bout with intense eccentric contractions was similar to the concentration found immediately after exercise, and still much lower than the resting level (15). In another study with a more moderate amount of eccentric exercise it was found that glycogen resynthesis was not impaired in the first 6 h after the exercise, but in the following 18 and 66 h (34).

In soccer the amount and intensity of eccentric exercise is without doubt less than in the studies cited above and the players are used to the exercise modes. Nevertheless, it is likely that some kind of muscle damage does occur during a soccer match due to eccentric exercise or physical contact during match-play. This damage might delay muscle glycogen resynthesis. It has been demonstrated that an increased ingestion of CHO can partially overcome the effect of the muscle damage on glycogen resynthesis (1). Thus, also in this respect the players can benefit from a high CHO intake following match play and training.

Summary

Soccer players should have a balanced diet that contains large amounts of carbohydrate to allow for a high training efficiency and for optimal preparation for matches. Therefore, it is important for the players to be conscious of the nutritive value of the food that they consume. The highest potential for storing glycogen in the muscles is immediately after exercise. It is therefore advisable to consume carbohydrate, either in solid or liquid form, shortly after a match or training session. This is particularly important if the players are training twice on the same day.

On the day of competition the last meal should be ingested three to four hours before the start, and it should mainly consist of carbohydrates that can be rapidly absorbed. During the last hour before a match, solid food or liquid with a high carbohydrate content may be avoided.

Fluid intake in soccer

In soccer the loss of body water, mainly due to the evaporation of sweat, can be large during competition. For example, under normal weather conditions the decrease in body fluid during a soccer match is approximately 2 l, and under extreme conditions the reduction in body water can be higher, e.g. in a World Cup soccer match in Mexico, one Danish player lost about 4.5 litres of fluid. Such changes in body fluid can influence performance negatively during match play (30). Thus, it is important for the players to take in fluid during a game and also during a training session to maintain the efficiency of the training. The question is what and how much to drink before, during and after training session or a game.

Before a training session or match

It is important that the players are not dehydrated before a match. The players should begin the process of "topping-up" with fluid already the day before a match. For example, an additional litre of juice can be drunk on the evening before a match, which will also provide an extra supply of sugar.

On the match-day, the players should have plenty to drink and be encouraged to drink even when they are not feeling thirsty. The content of sugar should be less than 10%. During the last hour before the match the players should not have more than 300 ml (a large cup) of a liquid with a sugar concentration less than 5% every 15 minutes. The intake of coffee should be limited as coffee contains caffeine, which has a diuretic effect and causes the body to lose a larger amount of water than is absorbed from the coffee.

During a training session or match

Besides reducing the net loss of body water, the intake of fluid can supply the body with carbohydrates. As low muscle glycogen concentrations in soccer might limit performance at the end of a match, intake of carbohydrate solutions during a match is useful.

Questions remain concerning the optimum composition of the drink, particularly with respect to its concentration, form of carbohydrates, electrolyte content, osmolality, pH, volume and temperature. These considerations depend, among other things, on the temperature and humidity of the environment, which should determine the ratio between the need for fluid and need for carbohydrates. In a cold environment there is a limited need for water, and a drink with a sugar concentration up to 10% can be used, whereas in a hot environment the carbohydrate content should be less than 5%. Before using drinks with high sugar concentrations in a match however, the players should have tried these drinks during training to ensure that stomach upset does not occur. There are large individual differences in the ability to tolerate drinks and to empty fluid from the stomach. While some players are unaffected by large amounts of fluid in the stomach, others find it difficult to tolerate even small quantities of fluid. The players will benefit by experimenting with different drinks and drinking habits during training. For further discussion of the compositions of the fluid see reference 25.

During a match small amounts of fluid should be drunk frequently. It is optimal to drink between 100 and 300 ml with a 2-5% sugar concentration every 10 to 15 minutes. In a soccer match, this will give a total fluid intake of between one and two litres, plus 30 to 50 grams of sugar during the match. This is sufficient to replace a significant amount of the water lost through sweat, and to cover some of the demand for carbohydrates. Although fluid intake during a match is important, it should not interfere with the game. The players should only drink when there is a natural pause in the game as the drinking may disturb the playing rhythm. It is convenient to place small bottles of fluid at different positions around the field in order to avoid long runs to the team bench.

After a training session or match

The players should drink plenty of fluid after a match and training. Several studies have demonstrated that restoration of fluid balance is a slow process and that it is not sufficient merely to increase fluid intake immediately after a match. It is not unusual that players are partially dehydrated on the day after a match. The body can only partially regulate water balance through the sensation of thirst as thirst is quenched before a sufficient amount of fluid has been drunk. Thus, in order to maintain fluid balance, more fluid has to be drunk than just satisfies the sensation of thirst.

The colour of urine is a good indicator of the fluid balance and the need for water. If the body is dehydrated, the amount of water in the urine is reduced and the colour becomes a stronger yellow.

Summary

The following recommendations regarding fluid intake may be helpful for a soccer player:
- Drink plenty of fluid the day before a match and on the day of the match – more than just to quench thirst.
- Drink frequently just before and during a match as well as at half-time, but only small amounts at a time – not more than 300 ml of fluid every 15 minutes.
- Drinks consumed just before and during a match should have a sugar concentration lower than 5% and a temperature between 5 and 10 °C.
- Drink a lot after a match – even several hours afterwards.
- Use the colour of the urine as an indication of the need for fluid – the yellower the urine, the greater the need for fluid intake.
- Experiment with drinking habits during training so that any difficulties in absorbing fluid during exercise can be overcome.

Acknowlegement

The studies performed by the author referred to in this review were supported by grants from Team Denmark and The Sport Research Council (Idrættens Forskningsråd).

References

1. Bak, J.F., Peterson, O. Exercise enhanced activation of glycogen synthase in human skeletal muscle. *Am J Physiol* 258, E957-E963, 1990.
2. Balsom, P.D. High intensity intermittent exercise: performance and metabolic responses with very high intensity short duration work periods. *Doctoral Thesis,* Karolinska Instituttet, Sweden, 1995.
3. Balsom, P.D., Ekblom, B., Söderlund, K, Sjödin, B., Hultman, E. Creatine supplementation and dynamic high-intensity intermittent exercise. *Scand J Med Sci Sports* 3, 143-149, 1993.
4. Balsom, P.D., Harridge, S.D.R., Söderlund, K., Sjödin, B, Ekblom, B. Creatine supplementation per se does not enhance endurance exercise performance. *Acta Physiol Scand* 149, 521-523, 1993.
5. Bangsbo, J. The physiology of soccer; with special reference to intense intermittent exercise. *Acta Physiol Scand* 151 (suppl. 160), 1-156, 1994.

6. Bangsbo, J. *Fitness Training for Football: A Scientific Approach*. HO + Storm, Brudelysvej 26A, 2880 Bagsværd, Denmark, 1994.

7. Bangsbo, J., Gollnick, P.D., Graham, T.E., Saltin, B. Substrates for muscle glycogen synthesis in recovery from intense exercise in humans. *J Physiol* 434, 423-440, 1991.

8. Bangsbo, J., Graham. T.E., Kiens, B., Saltin, B. Elevated muscle glycogen and anaerobic energy production during exhaustive exercise in man. *J Physiol.* 451, 205-222, 1992.

9. Bangsbo, J., Nørregaard, L, Thorsøe, F. The effect of carbohydrate diet on intermittent exercise performance. *Int J Sports Med* 13, 152-157, 1991.

10. Bergström, J., Hultman, E. Muscle glycogen synthesis after exercise: an enhancing factor localized to the muscle cells in man. *Nature* 210, 309-310, 1966.

11. Blom, P.C.S., Costill, D.L., Völlestad, N.K. Exhaustive running: inappropriate as stimulus of muscle glycogen supercompensation. *Med Sci Sports Exerc* 19, 398-403, 1987.

12 Blom, P.C.S., Hostmark, A.T., Vaage, O., Kardel, K. & Maehlum, S. Effect of different sugar diets on the rate of muscle glycogen synthesis. *Med Sci Sports Exerc* 19, 491-496, 1987.

13. Costill, D.L., Coyle, E.F., Dalsky, G., Evans, W., Fink, E. Hoppes, D. Effects of elevates plasma FFA and insulin on muscle glycogen usage during exercise. *J Appl Physiol* 43, 695-699, 1977.

14. Costill, D.L., Sherman, W.M., Fink, W.J., Maresh, C., Witten, M., Miller, J.M. The role of dietary carbohydrates in muscle glycogen resynthesis after strenous running. *Am J Clin Nutr* 34, 1831-1836.

15. Costill, D.L., Pascoe, D.D., Fink, W.J., Robergs, R.A., Barr, S.I., Pearson, D. Impaired muscle glycogen resynthesis after eccentric exercise. *J Appl Physiol* 69, 46-50, 1990.

16. Doyle, A.J, , Sherman, W.M. Eccentric exercise and glycogen synthesis. *Med Sci Sports Exerc* 23, 98S.

17. Essén, H. Studies on the regulation of metabolism in human skeletal muscle using intermittent exercise as an experimental model. *Acta Physiol Scand* 454, 1-32, 1978.

18. Gleeson, M., Maughan, R.J., Greenhaff, P.L. Comparison of the effects of pre-exercise feeding of glucose, glycerol and placebo on endurance and fuel homeostasis in man. *Eur J Appl Physiol* 55, 645-653, 1986.

19. Greenhaff, P.L., Bodin, K., Söderlund, I., Hultman, E. The effect of oral creatine supplementation on skeletal muscle phosphocreatine resynthesis. *Am J Physiol* 266, E725-E730, 1994.

20. Harris, R.S., Söderlund, K., Hultman, E. Elevation of creatine in resting and exercise muscles of normal subjects by creatine supplementation. *Clin Sci* 83, 367-374, 1992.

21. Ivy, J.L., Katz, A.L., Culter, C.L., Sherman, W.M., Coyle, E.F. Muscle glycogen synthesis after exercise: effect of time of carbohydrate ingestion. *J Appl Physiol* 64, 1480-1495, 1988.

22. Ivy, J.L., Lee, M.C., Brozinick, J.T., Reed, M.J. Muscle glycogen storage after different amounts of carbohydrate. *J Appl Physiol* 65, 2018-2023, 1988.

23. Jacobs, I., Westlin, N., Karlsson, J., Rasmusson, M., Haughton, B. Muscle glycogen and diet in elite soccer players. *Eur J Appl Physiol* 48, 297-302, 1982.

24. Kiens, B., Raben, A.B., Valeur, A.K., Richter, E.A. Benefit of dietary simple carbohydrates on the early postexercise muscle glycogen repletion in male athletes. *Med Sci Sports Exerc* 22, 588, 1990.

25. Maughan, R.J., Noakes, T.D. Fluid replacement and exercise stress. A brief review of studies on fluid replacement and some guidelines for the athlete. *Sports Med* 12, 16-31, 1991.

26. Neufer, P.D., Costill, D.L., Glynn, M.G., Kirwan, J.P. Mitchell, J.B., Houmard, J. Improvements in exercise performance: effects of carbohydrate feedings and diet. *J Appl Physiol* 62, 983-988, 1987.

27. Nordheim, K., Vøllestand, N.K., Glycogen and lactate metabolism during low-intensity exercise in man. *Acta Physiol Scand* 139, 475-484, 1990.

28. Piehl, K., Adolfsen, S, Nazer, K. Glycogen storage and glycogen synthetase activity in trained and untrained muscle of man. *Acta Physiol Scand* 90,779-788, 1974.

29. Plough, T., Galbo, H., Vingen, J., Jørgensen, M, Richter, E.A. Kinetics of glucose transport in rat muscle: effects of insulin and contractions. *Am J Physiol* 253, E12-E20, 1987.

30. Saltin, B. Aerobic work capacity and circulation at exercise in man: with special reference to the effect of prolonged exercise and/or heat exposure. *Acta Physiol Scand* (Suppl) 230, 1964.

31. Saltin, B. Metabolic fundamentals in exercise. *Med Sci Sports Exerc* 5, 137-146, 1973.

32. Sherman, W.M., Brodowicz, G., Wright, D.A., Allen W.K., Simonsen, J., Dernback, A. Effects of 4 h pre-exercise carbohydrate feedings on cycling performance. *Med Sci Sports Exerc* 21, 598-605, 1989.

33. Wagenmakers, A.J.M., Coakley, J.H., Edwards, R.H.T. Metabolism of branched-chain amino acids and ammonia during exercise: Clues from McArdle's disease. *Int J Sport Med* 11, 101-113, 1990.

34. Widrick, J., Costill, D.L., McConell, G.K., Anderson, D.E., Pearson, D.R., Zachwieja, J.J. Time course of glycogen accumulation after eccentric exercise. *J Appl Physiol* 75, 1999-2004, 1992.

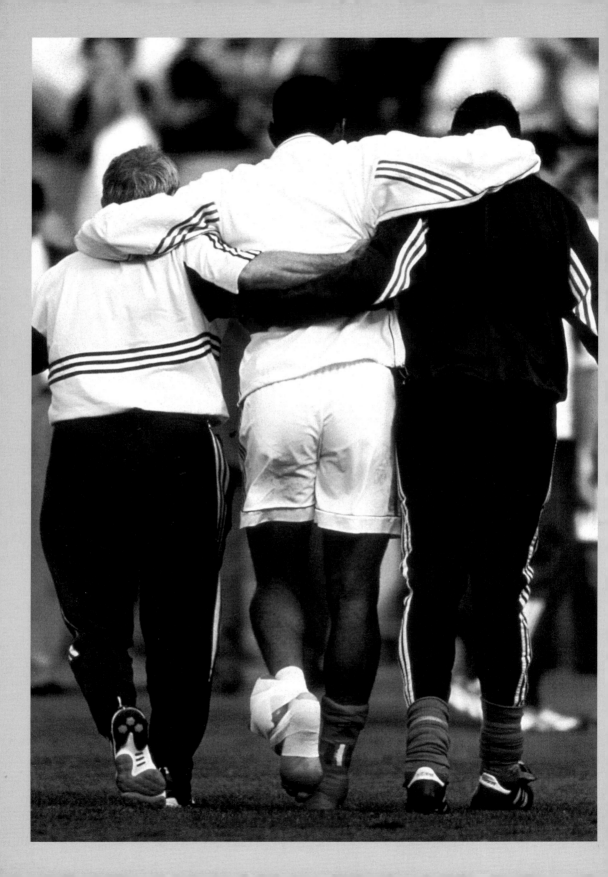

Injury Prediction In Soccer: Risk Factor Analysis

Han Inklaar

Synopsis

The aim of the study was to investigate if individual scores on internal and external risk factors in relationship with injuries add information to the aggregated team scores with respect to the risk of injury, taking the factors age group and level of play into account.

From a total population of 477 soccer players a non selective sample of 396 players was prospectively followed during the second half of the 1986/1987 competition. The sample was divided in two age groups (junior players, aged 13-19 years and senior players, aged 19 years and older) and in two levels of play. Eight internal risk factors and six external risk factors did not prove to be equally distributed over subgroups according to age and level of play. With four risk factors (number of injuries, frequency of practice, warming-up and age) 80% of the players could be predicted correctly with respect to their level of play.

For a high level of play the proportion of players injured was 23.9 ± 3.1 percent compared with 8.6 ± 2.3 percent for a low level of play. There was no difference in the risk of injury between the two age groups. Although univariately four risk factors (status of health, achievement motivation, warming-up, stretching) were associated with the risk of injury in matches, none of these variables contributed independly to the predictive value of the level of play in a logistic regression analysis. Based on individual observations with level of play the overall correct prediction of the risk of injury in matches *was 53% (48% non injured and 78% injured). With level of play 34% of the variance of the number of match injuries could be explained (F= 9.7, p <0.01).*

It is concluded that the variables used here add no information to the predictive value of the level of play with respect to the risk of match injuries. To our opinion the type of play associated with the level of play is an important predictor for match injuries in soccer. The higher the level of play, the rougher the type of play and the higher the risk of injury despite the more attention paid on preventive measures like practice, warming-up, cooling-down and stretching. Prevention primarily should be aimed at the behaviour of players during soccer matches. Adherence to the rules of the match is of utmost importance.

Introduction

The present literature on the epidemiology of soccer injuries shows conflicting data on the incidence, severity and aetiology of soccer injuries (19, 20). Different results may be partly explained by different definitions of injury and different methodological designs (19, 20).

Selection also may be responsible for different outcomes. Based on individual observations it has been demonstrated that the risk of injury is confounded by age and level of play.

In youth soccer the risk of injury increases with age (19). In senior soccer, on the contrary, the risk of injury decreases markedly above the age of 25 years (21). At a high level of play the risk of injury is much higher than the risk of injury at a low level of play (21, 24, 31). This difference appears to concern all age groups with exception of the 15/16 years age group (21). Injury rates on team scores also are not equally distributed over different age groups and levels of play (21). The level of play proved to be an important risk factor on the level of teams, strongly related to some injury characteristics. It is argued that the risk of injury primarily is related to teams, thereby suggesting, that this risk of injury outweighs the risk of injury for the individual player. In this study an attempt is made to present additional proof for this argumentation. On the level of individual players we will examine, if different scores on certain internal and external risk factors between individual players within teams may contribute to the explanation of the risk of injury. The current knowledge about risk factors for soccer injuries still is limited. The information is based on a number of cohort studies (20) and four randomised clinical trials (9, 22, 41, 45). The populations of study were selected homogenous subgroups of soccer players, mostly of a relatively high level of play. In the majority of the studies, the application of statistical analysis was restricted to descriptive and univariate analysing techniques. For male soccer players identified risk factors are: muscle tightness (7, 9, 26), muscle strength asymmetry (7, 9, 35), mechanical and functional instability (6, 11, 26, 30, 45), somatotype (38, 39), physical maturity (1, 39), maximal aerobic capacity (16), soccer skills (36, 39, 43, 48), behaviour (39) as internal risk factors and type of soccer activities (match, practice, warming-up, stretching) (8, 9, 13, 24, 31), the use of protective equipment (shinguards, ankle taping and bracing) (7, 9, 41, 45), shoe surface interrelation (7, 10, 29, 32, 44), opponent (7, 13, 31), rules of the match (7, 9, 13, 22, 31) as external risk factors.

The aim of this study therefore was to investigate if individual scores on internal and external risk factors in relationship with injuries add information to the aggregated team scores with respect to the injury risk, taking the factors age group and level of play into account. In other words, is it possible to detect differences of risk between individual players apart from risk scores related to teams, age groups and level of play?

Material and Methods

The members of two dutch non professional soccer clubs were prospectively followed during the second half of the 1986/1987 competition (February to June 1987). The population consisted of 245 senior players (aged over 18 years) and 232 junior players.

The senior players represented 17 teams of which for both clubs the first team was playing in the highest non professional division. The senior teams were divided into two levels of play. The first 3 teams of one club and the first 4 teams of the other club (together 101 players) were competing on a national (high) level; the other ten teams (144 players) were competing on a regional (low) level.

The junior players represented three age groups: 13-14 years, 15-16 years and 17-18 years. Each age group of youth players represented three teams per club. The combination of the first two teams of each group (for both clubs in total twelve teams ~ 156 players) was categorised as high level; the combination of the third teams of each age group (for both clubs six teams ~ 76 players) was categorised as low level.

Every week the players of each team had to report injuries sustained during official soccer activities (practice and matches) to a contact person delegated to the team. This weekly contact enabled us to follow the injured player with respect to medical treatment and absence from play. By weekly visits to both clubs virtually all reported injured players were examined by one of the authors. If necessary, additional information concerning diagnosis and medical treatment was obtained through phone calls to the general practitioner, specialist or physiotherapist of the injured player. The definition of injury was according to the definition accepted by the committee of experts in the project „Sports for all, sports injuries and their prevention" of the Council of Europe (46): „a soccer injury is a result of participation in official soccer activities resulting in a reduction in the amount or level of soccer activity, a need for advice or treatment and/or adverse social or economic effects".

Based on the soccer epidemiology literature a number of risk factors was selected for further analysis (Table 1). At the start of the study

Table 1. Selected risk factors for injury in soccer

Internal risk factors	External risk factors
age (yrs)	level of play
height (cm)	frequency of practice
body weight (kg)	duration of practice
percentage of body fat	warming-up
joint-mobility	cooling-down
muscle tightness	stretching
status of health	official rules violation
sports motivation	

players were invited to undergo biometry and to respond to question-naires with questions concerning the engagement in soccer, status of health and sports motivation. The biometry yielded the following inter-nal risk factors: height (cm), body weight (kg), sum of skinfolds (mm), joint mobility and muscle tightness. Skinfold measurements were accor-ding to the method of Durnin and Rahaman (4). The sum of 4 skinfold measurements (biceps, triceps, sub-scapular and suprailiacal) was used to estimate the percentage of body fat (4). Both factors were used in further analysis.

According to Lysens and coworkers (25) total joint mobility can be divided into three flexibility aspects i.e. active joint mobility, ligamen-tous laxity and muscle tightness.

The combination of these aspects with emphasis on active joint mo-bility and ligamentous laxity was measured by using the tests of joint-looseness validated by Marshall and coworkers (27). Thirteen joint-looseness tests were administered to non-injured joints of the upper and lower extremity. For each test a scale was constructed leading to the production of reliable measurements. The maximum score of the combination of the results on each test is 52. The sum of the test results is positively related to the joint-looseness.

The mobility of the back, hip as well as the flexibility of the ham-string muscles is measured in the sit and reach test[47]. In general the flexibility of the hamstring muscles pays the greatest contribution to the result of the test (17). Therefore this test was selected for the measure-ment of muscle tightness. The sit and reach test has a good test-retest reliability (23). The results are not influenced by body measures (3, 17, 28, 37, 42). There is a negative relation between the test result (cm) and the degree of muscle tightness (scores: 1= -20 till - 10 cm; 2= -10 till zero cm; 3= 0 - 10 cm; 4= 10 - 20 cm; 5= $ 20 cm).

Other internal risk factors used in this study are status of health and sports motivation.

The method of health screening through the use of a questionnaire was developed and tested by van Enst (14). The status of health is deter-mined by answers to questions regarding medical problems specifically related to sport. A positive answer to a question means a sports medical problem. A distinction can be made between questions with a B-qualification and questions with a C-qualification.

Regarding a positive answer to a B-question a sports medical advice is considered useful but not really necessary. A positive answer to a C-question implies the need for an urgent sports medical advice. Because there are several B-questions and C-questions the total B-score and/or total C-score may vary between persons. Here the status of health is only reflected by the total B-score (minor sports medical problems). The B-score especially concerns sports injury related questions in contrast to the C-score, which concerns more serious general sports related health problems. The higher the B-score, the worse the status of health is.

The sports motivation was reflected by four personality traits:
- achievement motivation, defined as the aim to achieve with respect to standards of excellence and to make efforts accordingly (15) (9 items, 5 answer categories).
- social affiliation i.e. the aim to obtain social experiences, contact and relation (15) (5 items, 5 answer categories).
- aggression i.e. to seek for tension and the risk for physical contact with the opponent, whether or not with the intention to injure him (15) (12 items, 5 answer categories).
- anxiety i.e. to discuss the feeling of self esteem by supposed impending or actual failure (40) (11 items, 3 answer categories).

Here, for soccer the questionnaire on motivation was developed and statistically validated by Pennings and Bol (34). To avoid empty cells in factorial analysis three point scales were used for each personality trait: achievement motivation (scores: 1= 0 - 30; 2= 31 - 35; 3= 36 - 45), social affiliation (scores: 1= 5 - 10; 2= 11 - 15; 3= 16 - 25), aggression (scores: 1= 5 - 25; 2= 25 - 30; 3= 31 - 56), anxiety (scores: 1= 11 - 15; 2= 15 - 20; 3= 21 - 30). A higher score means a more profound personality trait.

External risk factors used in this study were frequency and duration of practice, warming-up, cool-down, stretching and official rules violations.

The questions with respect to the engagement in soccer concerned:
- frequency of practice (scores: 1= never or less than once a week; 2= once a week; 3= twice a week; 4= three or more times a week)
- duration of practice (scores: 1= less than one hour a week; 2= 1 - 2 hours a week; 3= 2 - 3 hours a week; 4= 3 - 4 hours a week; 5= 4 or more hours a week)

- warming-up (scores: 1= no warming-up; 2= less than 10 minutes warming-up; 3= more than ten minutes warming-up)
- cooling-down (scores: 1= no cooling-down; 2= occasionally cooling-down; 3= yes, always cooling-down)
- stretching (scores: 1= no stretching; 2= yes, occasionally stretching; 3= yes, only every game stretching; 4= yes, every practice and game stretching)

Official rules violations resulting in an official warning or sending off the pitch were registered by the referee on the official game forms.

As to age a distinction was made between junior soccer players (13-19 years) and senior players (19 years and older).

As to level of play a distinction was made between high level of play (the first three or four senior teams and in each age category the first two junior teams) and low level of play (the remaining senior and junior teams).

The incidence of injury was defined as the number of injuries sustained in official soccer activities (match, practice) during the period of study. The risk of injury was expressed by the number of injuries per team.

Statistics

Because of social selection, based on the capacities and motivation of players and expectancies of coaches, internal and external risk factors of individual players were assumed to be highly related to the level of play. Therefore, firstly these risk factors were analysed univariately with regard to high and low level of play (Mann Whitney U-Wilcoxon Rank Sum W Test, SPSS). These analyses were based on individual scores.

Next, the relationships between individual risk scores and high versus low level of play were analysed multivariately in a logistic regression analysis.

The following step was to analyse the relationships between all risk factors (including scores on level of play) and the match injuries of individual players (zero = no injury, 1 = one or more match injuries). These analyses were performed univariately (Kruskal-Wallis one way analysis of variance).

Next, individual risk factor scores were used as predictors for the occurrence of game injuries. Hereto injured and non injured players were discriminated multivariately on the basis of logistic regression analysis.

Finally, all individual scores on risk factors, including level of play, were aggregated on the level of teams. Multiple regression analyes were used to establish, if other risk factor scores add to the explanation of the variance of the risk of injury by the level of play scores as obtained by logistic regression analysis.

The SPSS statistical package (33) was used for data analysis. The probability level accepted for statistical significance was set at $p < 0.05$.

Results

From the total population of 477 players 396 players underwent the biometry and responded to the questionnaires. With respect to the distribution over both levels of play and both age groups there was no difference between the sample of 396 players and the total population of soccer players (Table 2). However, with respect to the distribution

Table 2. Distribution of players and incident injuries from the total population and the sample over two age groups and two levels of play

	Total population N° of players N° of injuries		Sample N° of players N° of injuries	
Junior players				
low level	76	9	62	8
high level	156	34	132	30
Senior players				
low level	144	13	112	10
high level	101	27	90	24
Total	477	83	396	72

over both levels of play within the two age groups it was shown that in the sample of 396 players significant less players are registered in the subgroup of senior players acting at a low level of play (x^2= 4.51, df 3, 2-tailed p <0.05).

For the total population 75 out of 83 incident injuries were sustained during regular competition matches, of which 72 injuries were sustained in the sample (Table 2).

Using paired samples t-tests in none of the four subgroups according to age and level of play significant differences between the population and the sample could be demonstrated with respect to the number of game injuries in relation with the number of players in those subgroups. These analyses indicate that the sample of 396 players against the total population of 477 players was not selective.

Table 3 presents the median scores for every risk factor in relation to the level of play. Also further analyses were conducted to compare junior players and senior players with respect to the distribution of risk factors. The discriminating effect of the level of play on the distribution of the risk factors within these age groups also was examined. The data are not shown in a table, but significant results will be presented in the text.

Age
At a high level of play players were younger than players at a low level of play.

Biometry
At a high level of play players had less body weight than players at a low level of play.

However, this difference only was caused by differences in body weight found in the group of senior players. As to body fat a lower percentage was found at a high level of play. The difference in the percentage of body fat concerned both age groups. The combination of the results on body weight and body fat led to the conclusion that the difference in the lean body mass between players at a high level of play and a low level of play was markedly more pronounced in the senior age group. Senior players in general had more body fat than junior players (Z= -7.8, 2- tailed p= 0.000). Between both levels of play there was no difference in joint looseness . However, the performance on the sit and reach test was worse at a high level of play, suggesting

Table 3. Scores for risk factors by level of play (396 players)

risk factor	Low level of play			High level of play			Z	p-value
	median value	range	missing obser-vation	median value	range	missing obser-vation		
age (yrs)	25.21	39.15	0	17.92	40.47	0	- 7.3	***
height (cm)	177.00	45.50	0	178.00	54.50	14	- 0.2	NS
body weight (kg)	73.50	73.50	19	67.25	84.00	14	- 4.2	***
% body fat	16.30	23.60	19	11.75	18.80	14	- 6.3	***
joint-looseness	29.00	39.00	21	29.00	17.00	28	- 0.9	NS
sit and reach	3.00	4.00	19	3.00	4.00	14	- 2.1	*
B-score	1.00	7.00	0	1.00	7.00	0	- 0.2	NS
achievement motivation	1.00	2.00	34	2.00	2.00	15	- 6.6	***
agression	2.00	2.00	34	3.00	2.00	24	- 3.9	***
social affiliation	2.00	2.00	33	2.00	2.00	15	- 1.6	NS
anxiety	1.00	2.00	47	2.00	2.00	24	- 3.1	**
frequency of practice	2.00	3.00	0	3.00	3.00	0	- 9.7	***
duration of practice	2.00	4.00	13	3.00	4.00	1	-11.1	***
warming-up	2.00	2.00	0	1.00	2.00	0	- 9.2	***
cooling-down	3.00	2.00	0	3.00	2.00	0	- 2.6	**
stretching	2.00	3.00	0	1.00	3.00	0	- 8.6	***

significant differences between low and high level of play.
*** p <0.001, ** p <0.01, * p <0.05 (Mann Whitney U-Wilcoxon Rank Sum W Test, SPSS)

more hamstring muscle tightness. This difference in the performance on the sit and reach test only existed in the group of senior players (Z= -2.1, 2- tailed p <0.05). Senior players in general performed better on the sit and reach test than junior players (Z= -1.9, 2- tailed p= 0.05).

Status of health
Between both levels of play there was no difference in the score of minor sports related health problems. Senior players, however, reported more health problems than junior players (Z= -3.7, 2- tailed p <0.001).

Soccer motivation

At a high level of play players reported more achievement motivation. This difference was restricted to the group of senior players. Senior players in general was less motivated for achievement in soccer than junior players (Z= -3.6, 2- tailed p <0.001). The same picture was presented for agression. Also here senior players were less agressive than junior players (Z= -8.2, 2- tailed p= 0.000).

At a high level of play also more sports anxiety was reported. This difference between both levels of play concerned both age groups.

As to social affiliation no difference existed between both levels of play in the total sample.

However, within the subgroup of senior players at a low level of play significantly higher scores were found for the social affiliation than at a high level of play (Z= -2.22, 2- tailed p <0.05).

Soccer practice

Players at a high level of play reported to practise more frequently than players at a low level of play. This difference concerned both age groups. Senior players appeared to practice less frequently per week than junior players (Z= -3.4, 2- tailed p <0.001).

Warming-up, cooling-down, stretching

At a high level of play players reported in the questionnaire to spend more time on warming-up, cooling-down and stretching. For warming-up and stretching this difference concerned both age groups.

For cooling-down this difference only was noted in the group of senior players. In general senior players spent less time on warming-up (Z= -1.9, 2- tailed p= 0.05) and stretching (Z= -3.7, 2- tailed p <0.001) than junior players.

Prediction of level of play

The predictive value of risk factors with respect to the level of play was determined in a logistic regression analysis (method FSTEP LR). Four variables could be included in the equation: number of match injuries, frequency of practice, warming-up and age. The overall correct prediction with these variables was 80% (low level of play 83%, high level of play 77%). The exponent B values indicated that players at a high level of play practice more frequently, perform more warming-up, are younger and sustain more match injuries than players at a low level of play.

Injuries
For the total population of 477 players 115 players were registered with 46 prevalent and 83 incident injuries. Of the 83 incident injuries 57 injuries were sustained during regular competition matches, only 4 injuries during practice and 4 injuries during test matches. The overall incidence rate for teams was $17,5 \pm 2,2$ match injuries per 1000 playing hours. At a high level of play teams had a significant higher risk of injury in competition matches than teams at a low level of play ($22,6 \pm 2,8$ vs $11,4 \pm 2,9$ match injuries per 1000 playing hours, $F= 7,64$, $df= 1$, $p= 0.009$).

In the sample of 396 players 72 injuries were recorded, of which 68 injuries were sustained during matches (Table 2). At a high level of play significant more injuries were sustained than at a low level of play ($Z= -3.84$, 2- tailed $p= 0.0001$). The proportion of players injured in matches also was much higher at a high level of play than at a low level of play ($23.9 \pm 3.1\%$ injured versus $8.6 \pm 2.3\%$ injured, $Z= -3.78$, 2- tailed $p <0.001$).

With respect to the proportions of players injured in matches there was no difference between junior and senior players.

Prediction of match injuries
Until now the relationship between risk factors and the level of play was examined.

Next, the relationship between risk factors and the number of match injuries was examined. Again, individual scores on these variables were used.

Of the selected risk factors only the status of health ($x^2= 24.3$, $df = 5$, $p= 0.001$), achievement motivation ($x^2= 7.1$, $df = 5$, $p <0.05$), warming-up ($x^2= 18.4$, $df = 5$, $p= 0.0001$) and stretching ($x^2= 10.5$, $df = 7$, $p <0.05$) were associated with the risk of injury in games. The frequency of practice just failed to reach the level of significance ($x^2= 2.8$, $df = 7$, $p= 0.07$).

In a multivariate analysis (logistic regression analysis) non injured and injured players were discriminated on the basis of the individual scores on risk factors. With only the level of play the overall correct prediction was 53% (non injured players 48%, injured players 79%).

For the subgroup of senior players the overall correct prediction was 63% (non injured players 61%, injured players 76%). For the subgroup of junior players the overall correct prediction was 42% (non injured players 34%, injured players 79%). No other variables could be added to this model, meaning that the other risk factors do not change the picture obtained with the level of play.

The aggregation of the individual scores to teamscores of these variables may present a different picture. Therefore, the individually predicted values and residual values of the level of play, saved from the logistic regression analysis as well as the individual scores on other risk factors were aggregated to teamscores. Because each of these variables did not show any deviation from a standard normal distribution multiple regression analyses with the number of match injuries as a dependent variable could be applied. The team scores of match injuries in the sample were strongly related to the team scores of injuries per 1000 hours of play in the total population of 477 players ($r = .86$, $p < 0.001$). This justified the use of the aggregated team scores of match injuries as a dependent variable. Only the predicted and residual values of the level of play proved to be related to the aggregated number of match injuries (Multiple $R = .61$, adjusted $R^2 = .34$, $F = 9.7$, $p < 0.001$).

Discussion

The aim of this study was to demonstrate that in a heterogenous population of soccer players internal and external risk factors vary between soccer players from different age groups and different levels of play. Also we examined the level of play for its predictive value for the risk of injury in relation with the contribution of other risk factors.

The results indicate that many of the internal and external risk factors, measured here, are not equally distributed over two subgroups according to level of play. This unequal distribution sometimes concerned both age groups, and sometimes was restricted to one age group.

Biometry

The difference in body weight between both levels of play only was observed in the senior age group. Because in both age groups players at a high level of play had a lower percentage of body fat, it was concluded that the difference in lean body mass between players of a high level of play and players of a low level of play was markedly more pronounced in the senior age group. Between both levels of play as well as between both age groups there was no difference in joint-looseness. This underlined the conclusion of Marshall and co-workers (27) that joint-looseness is a trait of the person, here independent of age and level of play. No selection to the level of play took place on the basis of joint-looseness.

Senior players at a high level of play demonstrated a worse performance on the sit and reach test than senior players at a low level of play, suggesting more hamstring muscle tightness. This muscle tightness probably is caused by a higher load in practice and matches at a high level of play and not sufficiently compensated for by flexibility training. This finding is in agreement with the results of an other study (5), where soccer players of a relatively high level of play were compared with non soccer playing controls.

The fact that the group of junior players as a whole demonstrated more hamstring muscle tightness suggests the dominant influence of physical maturity with accerelated growth, resulting in a temporary discrepancy between skeletal growth and muscle growth.

Status of health

Selection towards the level of play obviously did not take place on the basis of the existence of minor sports related problems.

This finding is not remarkable, since in other studies (2, 5, 26, 31) of soccer players at a high level of play it was shown, that players in general tend to continue playing soccer despite the presence of minor injuries. Probably this relates to the culture in soccer to deny minor sports injuries as long as possible.

In senior players more minor sports related problems were reported. This result may be caused by an accumulation of minor and major injuries in the course of a soccer career. This history of soccer injuries may increase the probability of persisting complaints resulting from those injuries.

Soccer motivation

As might be expected at a high level of play players were more motivated for achievement and were more agressive. However, this difference between both levels of play only was noted in the group of senior players suggesting that selection towards level of play with respect to these risk factors takes places in the course of a lifetime.

The group of junior players as a whole expressed more achievement motivation and agression than the group of senior players. Maybe this is a general trait in the attitude of youth and not only related to soccer or sports in general, but also to other activities in our society. Extreme attitudes gradually will disappear during lifetime. As to sports anxiety the picture is different. At a high level of play in both age groups more sports anxiety was reported. Obviously, players at a high level of play have more difficulties in coping with the expectations of other persons (board, coach, fellow players, spectators) towards their performance in soccer. These problems in coping behaviour appear to persist in the course of the soccer career.

As to social affiliation only in the senior age group a difference was noted between both levels of play. This finding confirms our expectation that during a soccer career a progressive selection takes place. This selection is markedly more pronounced in senior soccer (12). Here players make their choice to quit soccer, or to play soccer only on a recreational basis with emphasis on sociability, or to continue playing soccer at a high level of performance, focusing on competition and the importance of winning.

Soccer practice

As might be expected players at a high level of play were practising more frequently and longer than players at a low level of play. The fact, that many senior teams at a low level of play did not practise at all, led to the conclusion, that senior players in general practise less frequently and with shorter duration of the practice than junior players.

Warming-up, cooling-down, stretching

At a high level of play players reported spending more time on warming-up, cooling-down and stretching. For cooling-down this difference only was noted in the group of senior players. Senior players in general spent less time on warming-up and stretching. Also here the more pronounced selection towards level of play in the senior age group may explain this finding. The senior soccer teams at a low level of play most often do not warm-up, stretch and cool-down at all.

Injuries

The vast majority of injuries in our study, as well as in other studies (8, 13, 24, 31, 36), were sustained in soccer matches. The risk of injuries in matches at a high level of play was about twice the risk of injuries in matches at a low level of play.

This finding is in agreement with the results of other studies (24, 31, 36).

Because we assumed that the level of play is an important risk factor for soccer injuries, the predictive value of the other risk factors with respect to the level of play was analysed. The level of play could be predicted well with four independent variables (number of match injuries, frequency of practice, warming-up and age). Univariately, only the status of health, achievement motivation, warming-up and stretching were associated with the risk of injury in matches.

However, in a logistic regression analysis only the level of play was shown to be of predictive value for the risk of injury in matches. With the level of play only the injured players could be predicted well. No other risk factor demonstrated an independent predictive value.

Based on our assumption that the risk of injury especially is related to the team, its characteristics and environment, also the predictive value of the teamscores of the selected risk factors was analysed.

Again only the level of play was shown to be related to the number of match injuries explaining 34% of the variance.

To our opinion it is the type of play, that differs between both levels of play and even between teams on the same level of play. The increased importance of the results of competition matches at a high level of lay most likely will result in more risk taking behaviour and a more rough character of the match. Support for this assumption is obtained by the analysis of rules violations. For example, in our study significant more official rules violations were registered at a high level of play ($Z= -1.9$, one tailed p <0.05). However, this difference between both levels of play only exists in the group of senior players ($Z= -3.5$, one tailed p <0.001). To our opinion the group of junior players as a whole still is rather homogenous. This is reflected by the soccer motivation, showing no difference between the two levels of play with respect to achievement motivation and agression. In the group of junior players selection to-wards level of play only starts to take place, but in the group of senior players the process of selection almost has been completed resulting in two levels of play, markedly different from each other. At a low level of play senior players still are active in soccer because of sociability. The type of play is adjusted accordingly with few injuries and official rules violations. At a high level of play competition is the important issue, resulting in a hard type of play with more injuries and official rules violations. With respect to the official rules violations our finding is supported by van Galen (18), who showed the status of the referee and the division level to be the most important discriminating varia-bles between 1750 matches with and 1750 matches without disciplinary cases in non professional soccer. Together with the goal difference, the phase of soccer season and the geographical distance between two clubs these variables could explain 15% of the variance of matches with disciplinary cases. An official referee, a high level of play, a small goal difference, the start of the soccer season and a small distance be-tween both clubs are associated with a higher risk of matches with disciplinary cases.

Although the level of play seems the most important predictor for the risk of injury, even between teams acting on the same level of play the risk of injury may differ considerably.

This difference is caused by the difference in the type of play and the environment of a team. For example, Schmikli (39) applied observa-tional analysis to 115 matches of 13-16 years old junior players.

The results showed that corrected for teams actions of players toget-her with the quality of a warming-up and the age group were signifi-cantly (p= 0.000) related to the number of injuries per team, explaining 65.8% of the variance in this injury rate. Actions contributing to the risk of injury were tripping, blocking tackles, kicking and stamping of the opponent. These actions again suggest a rough character of an injury prone match. Also other predictor variables may be taken into consideration. For example, Wisman (48) examined the relation between time scores of two ball skill tests and the average number of injuries per player in a group of 82 soccer players, aged 11-17 years. The scores of both tests significantly (R= .69, p <0.01 and R= .68, p <0.05) were related to the average number of injuries explaining 23% of the variance of injury.

Finally, it is notewortly that prevalent injuries do not have a predictive value for the risk of injury. This finding supports our idea, that it is mainly coincidental which player gets injured within a team.

In conclusion, the results in our study seem to be rather contradictory. Teams of players that practise more frequently and longer and perform more warming-up and stretching, show a higher risk of injury in matches. However, selection towards the level of play and the associated type of play here are the confounding variables, with a higher incidence of match injuries and official rules violations at a high level of play.

The more selection towards the level of play, the rougher the type of play and the higher the risk of injury is. This may explain the high injury rate noted in professional soccer (2, 13, 26). Finally, it should be emphasized that the small number of soccer teams (n= 35), the rather small number of incident injuries and the interaction with the confounding variables age and level of play limited the power of statistics in our study and prevented a thorough statistical analysis within the different subgroups.

Recommendations

To our opinion primary prevention mainly has to focus on the behaviour of players during the matches of teams acting on relatively high levels of play. Attention should be paid to the selection and training of the official referees. The best referees should be appointed to matches, where difficult circumstances may be expected. Adherence to the rules hereby is of utmost importance. Also good ball skills at high speed as well as a well conducted warming-up may diminish the risk of injury. Secondary prevention (first aid, medical diagnosis, treatment and rehabilitation) predominantly should be directed to teams acting on relatively high levels of play. In terms of profits and losses this approach seems to be most profitable for the health care in soccer. Future studies are necessary to support our point of view, preferably repeating our approach within homogenous subgroups of soccer players.

Acknowledgements

The study was financially supported by the former Dutch Ministry of Welfare, Public Health and Cultural Affairs (now called Dutch Ministry of Public Health, Welfare and Sport) and by the former National Institute for Sports Health Care.

References

1. Backous D.D., Friedl K.E., Smith N.J., Parr Th.J., Carpine W.D.: *Soccer Injuries and their relation to physical maturity.* Am. J. Dis. Child. 142, 839-842, 1988
2. Becker G.: *Sportverletzungen und Sportschäden bei Berufsfussballspielern.* Dissertation Joh. Gutenberg University, Mainz, 1987
3. Broer M.R., Galles N.R.G.: *Importance of relationship between various body measurements in the performance of the toe-touch test.* Research Quarterly 29, 253-263, 1958
4. Durnin J.V. Rahaman M.H.: *Body fat assessed from total body density and its estimation from skinfold thickness.* Br. J. Nutr. 21, 681-689, 1967
5. Ekstrand J.: *Soccer injuries and their prevention.* Linköping University, medical dissertation. Linköping, no 130, 1982
6. Ekstrand J., Gillquist J.: *Soccer injuries and their mechanisms: a prospective study.* Med. Sci. Sports Med. Exerc. 15, 3, 267-270, 1983
7. Ekstrand. J., Gillquist J.: *The avoidability of soccer injuries.* Int. J. Sports Med. 4, 124-128, 1983
8. Ekstrand J., Gillquist J., Möller M. et al. *Incidence of soccer injuries and their relation to training and team success.* Am. J. Sports Med. 11, 63-67, 1983
9. Ekstrand J., Gillquist J., Liljedahl S.O.: *Prevention of soccer. Supervision by doctor and physiotherapist.* Am. J. Sports Med. 11, 116-120, 1983
10. Ekstrand J., Nigg B.: *Surface related injuries in soccer.* Sports Med. 8, 56-62, 1989
11. Ekstrand J., Tropp H.: *Incidence of ankle sprains in soccer.* Foot Ankle 11, 1, 41-43, 1990
12. Ekstrand J., Roos H., Tropp H.: *Normal course of events amongst Swedish soccer players: an 8- year follow-up study.* Br. J. Sp. Med. 24, 2, 117-119, 1990
13. Engström B., Forssblad M., Johansson C. et al: *Does a major knee injury definitely sideline an elite soccer player?* Am. J. Sports Med. 18, 101-105, 1990

14. Enst van G.C.: *De ontwikkeling van een selectiemethode in het periodiek preventief sportmedisch onderzoek. (Engl. summary)* Thesis, University of Amsterdam, 1990

15. Erdmann R.: Motiventwicklung als Lernprosz. *In: Erdmann R. (Ed.): Motive und Einstellungen im Sport.* Karl Hoffman. Verlag, Schorndorf, 1983

16. Eriksson L.I., Jorfeldt L., Ekstrand J.: *Overuse and distorsion soccer injuries related to the players estimated maximal aerobic work capacity.* Int. J. Sports Med. 7, 214-216, 1986

17. Fieldman H.: *Relative contribution of the back and hamstrings muscles in the performance of the toe-touch test after selected extensibility excercises.* Research Quarterly 39, 518-523, 1968

18. Galen van W.Ch.: *Overtredingen en strafzaken in het amateurvoetbal. (Engl. summary).* Thesis University of Limburg, Maastricht, 1986

19. Inklaar H.: *Soccer Injuries I: Incidence and Severity.* Sports Med. 18, 1, 55073, 1994

20. Inklaar H.: *Soccer Injuries II: Aetiology and Prevention.* Sports Med. 18, 2, 81-93, 1994

21. Inklaar H., Bol E., Schmikli S. Mosterd W.L.: *Injuries in male soccer players: team risk analysis.* Submitted for publication

22. Jörgensen U., Sörensen J.: Free substitution in soccer: A prospective study. *In: Togt van der C.R., Kemper A.B.A., Koornneef M., editors. Proceedings 3rd Meeting Council of Europe. Sports injuries and their prevention.* National Institute for Sports Health Care, Oosterbeek, 155-158, 1988

23. Kemper H.C.G., Verschuur R.: *Moper-fitness test lichamelijke prestatie geschiktheidstest voor de lichamelijke opvoeding.* Richting 31, 2-6, 22-25, 1977

24. Latella F., Serni G., Aglietti P., Zaccherotti G., De Biase P.: *The epidemiology and mechanisms of soccer injuries.* J. Sports Traumatol. 14, 2, 107-117, 1992

25. Lysens R.J.J., Lefevre J., Ostijn M.S., Brodie D.A.: *Study of evaluation of joint flexibility as a risk factor in sports injury.* The Cilag Award of the Belgian Society of Sports Medicine and Sports Science University Press, Leuven, 1984

26. Lysens R.J.J.: Epidemiological study of soccer injuries in the 18 teams of the first national division of the Royal Belgium Soccer Association (RBSA) during the season 1980-1981. *In: Togt van der C.R., Kemper A.B.A., Koornneef M., editors. Proceedings 2nd Meeting Council of Europe: Sports injuries and their prevention.* National Institute for Sports Health Care, 16-17, 1987

27. Marshall J.L., Johanson N., Wickiewicz Th. L. et al: *Joint Looseness: A function of the person and the joint.* Med. Sci. Sports Exerc. 12, 189-194, 1980

28. Mathews D.K., Shaw V., Woods J.B.: *Hip flexibility of elementary school boys as related to body segments.* Research Quarterly 30, 297-305, 1959

29. Monto R.R.: *Time to redesign the trusty football boot?* New Scientist, 4, 15, 1993

30. Neyret P., Donell S.T., Dejour D., Dejour H.: *Partial meniscectomy and anterior cruciate ligament rupture in soccer players.* Am. J. Sports Med. 3, 21, 455-460, 1993

31. Nielsen A., Yde J.: *Epidemiology and traumatology of injuries in soccer.* Am. J. Sports Med. 17, 6, 803-807, 1989

32. Nigg B.M., Segesser B.: *The influence of playing surface on the load on the locomotor system and on football and tennis injuries.* Sports Med. 5, 375-385, 1988

33. Norusis M.J.: *SPSS/PC+ Advanced Statistics,* Chicago, Illinois, SPSS Inc., 1986

34. Pennings A.H., Bol E.: *Motivationele Oriëntaties bij Spelers in het Amateurvoetbal.* Internal publication Janus Jongbloed Research Centre, University of Utrecht, Utrecht, 1987

35. Poulmedis P.: Muscular imbalance and strains in soccer. *In: Togt van der C.R., Kemper A.B.A., editors. Proceedings 3rd Meeting Council of Europe.* Sports injuries and their prevention. National Institute for Sports Health Care, Oosterbeek, 53-57, 1988

36. Poulsen T.D., Freund K.G., Madsen F., Sandvej K.: *Injuries in high-skilled and low-skilled soccer: A prospective study.* Br. J. Sp. Med. 25, 3, 151-153, 1991

37. Renson R., Ostyn M., Simons J. et al: *Studie over de physical fitness bij school-gaande jongens van 12- tot 19- jarige leeftijd. Struktuur van de lenigheid en faktoren die haar bepalen.* Hermes, Tijdschr. Inst. Lich. Opl. Leuven, 6, 215-225, 1972.

38. Salokun S.O.: *Minimizing injury rates in soccer through preselection of players by somatotypes.* J. Sports Med. Phys. Fitness, 34, 64-69, 1994

39. Schmikli S.L.: *Blessures in jeugdvoetbal.* Publication Department of Medical Physiology and Sports Medicine, University of Utrecht, 1994.

40. Schwenkmezger P.: Schwerpunkte der Angstforschung in Psychologie und Sportpsychologie. *In: Janssen J.P. & Hahn E. (ED.): Aktivierung Motivation, Handlung und Coaching im Sport.* Karl Hofmann Verlag, Schorndorf, 1983

41. Surve I., Schwellnus M.P., Noakes T., Lombard C.: *A Fivefold Reduction in the Incidence of Recurrent Ankle Sprains in Soccer Players Using the Sport-Stirrup Orthosis.* Am. J. Sports Med. 5, 22, 601-606, 1994

42. Swalus P.: *Bijdrage tot de studie der relaties tussen de houding enerzijds, het somatotype, de lenigheid en de kracht anderzijds.* Hermes, Tijdschr. Inst. Lich. Opl. Leuven, 2, 219-226, 1967/1968

43. Taimela S., Österman L., Kujala U.M., et al.: *Motor ability and personality with reference to soccer injuries.* J. Sports Med. Physical Fitness 30, 2, 194-201, 1990

44. Torg J.S., Quedenfeld T.: *Effect of shoe type and cleat length on incidence and severity of knee injuries among high school football players.* Res. Q. 42, 2, 203-211, 1971

45. Tropp M., Asking C., Gillquist J.: *Prevention of ankle sprains.* Am. J. Sports Med. 13, 259-262, 1985

46. Vulpen van A.V.: *Sports for all, sports injuries and their prevention, scientific report.* Council of Europe, Oosterbeek, National Institute for Sports Health Care, 1989

47. Wells K.F., Dillon E.K.: *The sit and reach test of back and leg flexibility.* Research Quarterly 23, 115-118, 1952

48. Wisman J.G.J.: *Voetbalvaardigheden en Blessurerisico.* Internal Publication Department of Medical Physiology and Sports Medicine, University of Utrecht, 1991.